T0297728

THE VISUAL BRAIN
 Peripheral Reading and Writing Disorders

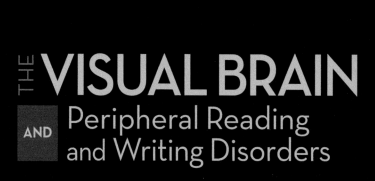

THE VISUAL BRAIN
AND Peripheral Reading and Writing Disorders

Heidi McMartin Heeringa, MS, CCC-SLP

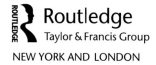

Routledge
Taylor & Francis Group

NEW YORK AND LONDON

First published 2019 by SLACK Incorporated

Published 2024 by Routledge
605 Third Avenue, New York, NY 10158

and by Routledge
4 Park Square, Milton Park, Abingdon, Oxon OX14 4RN

Routledge is an imprint of the Taylor & Francis Group, an informa business

Cover Artist: Christine Seabo

Library of Congress Cataloging-in-Publication Data

Names: Heeringa, Heidi McMartin, author.
Title: The visual brain and peripheral reading and writing disorders : a
   guide to visual system dysfunction for speech-langauge pathologists /
   Heidi McMartin Heeringa.
Description: Thorofare, NJ : Slack Incorporated, 2019. | Includes
   bibliographical references and index.
Identifiers: LCCN 2019007526 (print) | ISBN 9781630915414 (paperback)
Subjects: | MESH: Visual Perception | Language Disorders--diagnosis | Visual
      Pathways | Vision, Ocular | Language Disorders--therapy Classification: LCC RC423 (print) | NLM
                                                                                              WW 105 | DDC
   616.85/5075--dc23
LC record available at https://lccn.loc.gov/2019007526

ISBN: 9781630915414 (pbk)
ISBN: 9781003526919 (ebk)

DOI: 10.4324/9781003526919

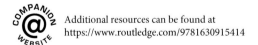

Additional resources can be found at
https://www.routledge.com/9781630915414

DEDICATION

This book is dedicated to Betty Jane McMartin (1923-2011) for your commitment to the fields of occupational therapy and special education.

Thank you to WC, LM, DS, and HW for sharing your insights into acquired dyslexia and dysgraphia.

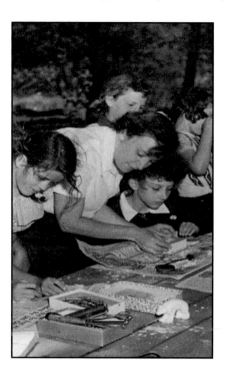

CONTENTS

ABOUT THE AUTHOR

Heidi McMartin Heeringa, MS, CCC-SLP is a speech-language pathologist with 36 years experience working with adult clients with dysphagia, aphasia, apraxia, and cognitive-communicative dysfunction in the rehabilitation setting. Acquired reading disorders and the relationship between visual system dysfunction and cognitive-communicative function are areas of special interest and expertise. The author holds a bachelor's degree in linguistics and master of science in speech-language pathology from the University of Michigan. Other publications by this author include *A Manual for the Treatment of Reading and Writing Disorders* (2002) and the *Assessment of Language-Related Functional Activities* (Baines, Martin, & McMartin Heeringa, 1999).

INTRODUCTION

In my work as a speech-language pathologist, I have been puzzled by client statements such as "I can see the clock, but I don't know where it is," or "If I take my eyes off the pencil tip, I don't know where I am," or "I'm having an awful time reading. I'm spending too much time figuring out what a letter is." Reading and writing are frequently impaired following stroke and traumatic brain injury (Thiagarajan, Ciuffreda, Ludlam, 2011). Neurological disorders frequently produce changes in visual system function that result in the inability to orient oneself or localize objects in space, or recognize or sequence visual forms including objects, letters, and words. The working memory components of reading and writing such as the ability to maintain the mental image of words (visual spatial sketchpad) and the ability to use inner speech (phonological buffer) to refresh the auditory trace of letter names, numbers, and words while we spell, take notes, or make a phone call, may be negatively impacted by injury to the brain. These changes can have a profound impact on functional communication, learning, and functional independence.

According to Wolf (2007), three principles of brain organization form the foundation of our ability to learn to read: "the capacity to make new connections among (evolutionary) older structures; the capacity to form areas of exquisitely precise specialization for recognizing patterns in information; and the ability to learn to recruit and connect information from these areas automatically." Reading and writing engage central language skills such as knowledge of phonetics, vocabulary, and grammar; prelexical (peripheral) sensory skills such as color, contrast sensitivity, and form recognition; the oculomotor skills of fixation, saccades, and convergence; and access to graphomotor programs for printing and writing. When we read and write, the early bottom-up visual processes that lead to letter and word recognition and written spelling are integrated with central language processes such as phonological awareness and the top-down cognitive processes of visual attention and memory. Visual sensory and visual motor deficits interfere with bottom-up visual processes, leading to various acquired reading and writing disorders.

My purpose for writing this text was to: broaden my own understanding of how visual sensory and visual motor impairments lead to peripheral reading and writing disorders, and how they differ from central language disorders such as aphasia; and identify treatment methods that are best suited to clients with peripheral visual language dysfunction. Chapter 1 reviews the fundamental visual processes involved in reading and writing. Chapter 2 describes how these processes may be affected by aging, stroke, brain injury, or progressive neurological disease. Methods for incorporating this knowledge into the practice of speech-language pathology are provided in Chapter 3. Treatment suggestions that capitalize on the visual system's potential for functional recovery are based on: an extensive literature review in the areas of normal and disordered visual function, and the relationship between vision, language, and cognition; consultation within the fields of neuro-optometry and occupational therapy; and continuing education in the area of visual system impairments and brain injury—as well as 36 years of experience in the field of speech-language pathology and the treatment of neurogenic cognitive-communicative disorders. By addressing visual system impairments as part of the rehabilitation process, we can achieve better outcomes in adult clients with peripheral reading and writing disorders and cognitive-communicative dysfunction. For a comprehensive text on normal and disordered visual function in children and its impact on language and reading, the reader is referred to Zihl and Duther's 2015 book cited at the end of this introduction.

—*Heidi McMartin Heeringa, MS, CCC-SLP*

REFERENCES

Thiagarajan, P., Ciuffreda, K. J., & Ludlam, D. P. (2011). Vergence dysfunction in mild traumatic brain injury (mTBI). *Ophthalmologic and Physiological Optics, 31,* 456-468.

Wolf, M. (2007). *Proust and the squid: The story and science of the reading brain* (p. 12). New York, NY: HarperCollins Publishers.

Zihl, J., and Duther, G. N. (2015). *Cerebral visual impairments in children: Visuoperceptive and visuocognitive disorders.* Wien, Austria: Springer-Verlag.

1

Anatomy of the Eye and Visual Brain

Vision is more than seeing. It is our primary source of sensory information and plays a major role in cognition, language, and action. Vision involves the integration of sensory information relating to form, color, location, and temporal sequence with input from other sensory systems (e.g., auditory, tactile, proprioceptive, kinesthetic) (Helvie, 2011; Sanet & Press, 2011). The ability to group these elements and bind them together is the key to our ability to recognize objects, read, and write. Sensory components of the visual system continuously change light stimuli into recognizable forms that are organized spatially and temporally and associated with previously learned knowledge of objects, space, and actions. This process begins in the retina and advances through various cortical and subcortical structures. Auditory, visual, and somatosensory neural pathways project sensory information to the thalamus where it is transmitted throughout the central nervous system. Auditory and visual sensory input are integrated in the midbrain and are necessary to our sense of spatial orientation and balance (Okoye, 1997). Topographical organization of sensory input preserves information on the location of visual stimuli for all visually-mediated activities.

Speech-language pathologists frequently instruct clients to look, read, match, talk, and write about object, picture, and word stimuli. Locating objects in relation to ourselves (i.e., egocentric localization) requires the integration and continuous updating of input from the visual-sensory system with input on head and eye position from the vestibular and proprioceptive systems (Dutton, 2003; Helvie, 2011). Likewise, in order to manipulate objects and/or to scan and interpret a series of objects such as words in a sentence, we need to be able to locate one object or word in relation to another (allocentric localization) (Dijkerman, Milner, & Carey, 1998; Grainger & Holcomb, 2009; Halligan, Fink, Marshall, & Vallar, 2003; Reinhart, Schindler, & Kerkhoff, 2011). Visual language processing also relies on the ability to maintain steady gaze long enough to process visual detail, and the ability to shift the focus of visual attention to scan pictures or sentences. In this chapter, we will review the structural elements of the eye, the cortical and subcortical structures, and the motor and sensory components of vision in the human brain.

McMartin Heeringa, H. *The Visual Brain and Peripheral Reading and Writing Disorders: A Guide to Visual System Dysfunction for Speech-Language Pathologists*. (pp. 1-22).
© 2019 Taylor & Francis Group.

STRUCTURAL COMPONENTS OF THE EYE

The eye is composed of a lens system at the front and the photosensitive retina at the back. For an illustration of the anatomy of the orbit and retina the reader is referred to Hubel (1995). The cornea and sclera form the external layer of the eye. The cornea is a transparent cover over the pupil and iris. It has no pigment or blood vessels. The curved surface of the cornea refracts light rays directing them to the retinal photoreceptors. The sclera is the white part of the eye. Its opaque quality keeps light from entering the eye to reduce glare. Six pairs of extraocular muscles connect the sclera to the skull and move the eyes horizontally, vertically, and diagonally. Cranial nerves (CNs) III, IV, and VI innervate these muscles (Gillen, 2009).

The pupil is the central opening in the iris, which is the colored portion of the eye. Two muscles control the size of the pupil to allow more or less light into the eye: the dilator muscle increases the pupil size, while the iris sphincter muscle reduces the pupil opening to limit the amount of light that enters the orbit (Schiff, 1997). The translucent lens works with the iris to achieve a sharp, focused image on the retinal photoreceptors. The ciliary body sits behind the iris and is composed of the ciliary muscle and ciliary processes that connect to the lens. Muscle contractions of the ciliary body change the shape of the lens for viewing objects both near and far. When viewing near objects the lens has a more spherical shape while it becomes flatter for viewing objects at a distance (Hubel, 1995). The retina is a multi-layered, light-sensitive area of the eye. It contains four different types of neurons: bipolar, ganglion, horizontal, and amacrine cells. Rods and cones are photoreceptors found in the outermost sensory layer of the retina. Rods in the peripheral retina respond to low light and movement in the peripheral visual field. Rods are not sensitive to color; thus, we are colorblind in dim light (Farah, 2000). Bright light- and color-sensitive cones are located in the central retina, also called the *fovea* (Hubel, 1995; Zeki, 1993). Color vision is dependent upon the response of cone cells to bright light. When we fixate on objects of interest the image is projected directly onto the fovea where cone cells are most densely concentrated.

The first synapse of the visual pathway occurs in the retina between the rods and cones of the outer sensory layer and the bipolar cells of the second layer. The horizontal and bipolar cells of the second retinal layer contribute to the perception of color, contrast, and brightness. These cells then synapse with the retinal ganglion cells (Farah, 2000; Webb & Adler, 2007). At this early level of visual processing a retinal map is formed that codes any retinal point where a lighter area meets a darker area across the entire visual field (Farah, 2000). This contrast sensitivity is necessary for form recognition (see page. 10 for more detail). In a review of 20 years of research on reading and eye movement patterns, neuropsychologist Keith Rayner (1998) divided the retina into three distinct areas: the fovea or central one to three degrees where focal vision is most acute; the parafovea ranging five degrees on either side of the fovea; and the peripheral retina outside the parafovea (Figure 1-1). These distinctions are important in a later discussion of reading in Chapter 2.

The processing of visual-sensory input and the motor control of ocular muscles involve CNs II, III, IV, and VI; brainstem structures; optic tract; lateral geniculate nucleus (LGN) a complex, six-layered structure that forms part of the cortical thalamus; and the striate (primary visual) and prestriate (visual association) cortexes in the occipital lobe. The optic nerve (CN II) is formed by about 1 million retinal nerve cells exiting each eye at the optic disk or blind spot. The point at which the two optic nerves meet and cross is called the *optic chiasm* (Figures 1-2, 1-5). Beyond the optic chiasm, optic nerve fibers carry input from the right and left peripheral visual fields to the contralateral hemisphere. Optic fibers that do not cross over provide input from the central visual fields to the ipsilateral hemisphere (Rayner, 1998; Zeki, 1993). When a word is fixated, letters that fall to the left of midline are processed by the right hemisphere, and letters that fall to the right of midline are processed by the left hemisphere (Whitney & Lavador, 2004). Letters are then bound into word forms at the cortical level.

Neighboring retinal ganglia are grouped together in the optic nerve (CN II). In the early stages of visual processing they send information about motion, color, line orientation, and direction

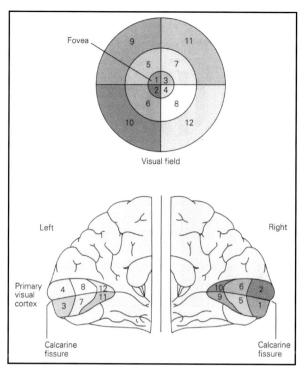

Figure 1-1. Each half of the visual field is represented in the contralateral primary visual cortex. In humans, the primary visual cortex is located at the posterior pole of the cerebral hemisphere and lies almost exclusively on the medial surface. Areas in the primary visual cortex are devoted to specific parts of the visual field, as indicated by the corresponding numbers. The upper fields are mapped below the calcarine fissure and the lower fields above it. The striking aspect of this map is that about half of the neural mass is devoted to representation of the fovea and the region just around it. This area has the greatest visual acuity. (Reprinted with permission from Kandel, E. R., Schwartz, J. H., & Jessel, T. M. [2000], *Principles of neural science* [4th ed]. New York, NY: McGraw-Hill Education.)

through the optic chiasm and optic tract to the LGN (Figures 1-2 and 1-3) where 90% of optic fibers end (Kandel, Schwartz, & Jessel, 1995; Tong, 2003). The LGN regulates, relays and filters input to and from multiple areas of the cortex including the primary visual cortex and the visual association cortex (Baker, 2000). Cells of the LGN, just like the retinal ganglia, are sensitive to contrast (Zeki, 1993). The central visual field is more generously represented in the retina, optic tract, and cortex than the peripheral fields (Baker, 2000; Kandel et al., 1995; Schneider, Richter, & Kastner, 2004). In the visual system, just as in the motor and sensory systems, the flow of information occurs in both a parallel and sequential manner. For an excellent illustration of this process the reader is referred to Danckert and Rosetti (2005) or Diedrich, Stebbins, Schlitz, and Goetz (2014).

Prior knowledge of objects and actions on objects is integrated with current visual input. This begins with basic feature analysis and continues on to more complex analysis of objects and scenes (Mesulam, 1998; Wolf, 2007). Buonomano and Merzenich (1998) describe the flow of visual information as follows: "… at each level of processing, the neurons are sampling from a larger input space, receiving convergent information from the previous level, diverging out to the next level, and in the process, forming larger and more complex integrated and combinatorial receptor fields." As visual sensory input travels from the retina to the cortex, it is segregated by the eye of origin and organized topographically (Hubel, 1995; Zeki, 1993). In *Proust and the Squid: The Story and Science of the Reading Brain*, Maryanne Wolf (2007) states that due to retinotopic organization "… every line, diagonal, circle or arc seen by the retina in the eye activates a specific, specialized location in the occipital lobes in a split second." Topographical mapping of spatial information in the visual pathways is consistent with the organization of the somatosensory, auditory, and motor systems (Kandel, 2006). These topographic, tonotopic, and retinotopic maps can change across the lifespan in response to learning (Buonomano & Merzenich, 1998) and to changes that result from motor and sensory system dysfunction. This neuroplastic change occurs at the synaptic level based on disease, brain injury, experience, or therapeutic intervention (Kelly, Foxe, & Garavan, 2006; Ludlow et al., 2008).

THE ROLE OF THE BRAINSTEM IN VISION

The brainstem is located between the cerebral hemispheres and the spinal cord. The midbrain of the brainstem receives 10% of all visual input through the retinotectal pathway (Kandel et al., 1995; Tong, 2003). The peripheral retina is indicated by numbers 9, 10, 11 and 12 in Figure 1-1. The retinotectal pathway provides visual input from the peripheral retina to the superior colliculi (SC), multi-layered structures that form part of the roof (tectum) of the midbrain (de Gelder, 2010; Ro & Rafal, 2006). The SC control pupil constriction and determine the amount of light entering the eye (Hammond, 2000; Kandel et al., 1995). They also regulate the amount of eye, head, and body movement needed to take in visual stimuli, locate objects and reach for them (Baker, 2000; Okoye, 1997). The SC contain a topographical motor map that directs attention while controlling eye movements that place visual stimuli at the fovea (Farah, 2000; Sanet & Press, 2011). Saccades are the quick eye movements that center objects of our attention on the fovea (Greenlee, 2003). As we read a single page of text, hundreds of saccades alternate with fixations to bring letters and words to our attention (Rayner, 1998) while filtering out other visual stimuli. These well-coordinated eye movements and sustained fixations at precise locations are essential to the reading process and near language activities including writing, computer use, and instrumental activities of daily living (Gillen, 2009).

All visual areas of the brain have projections to the SC including the retina, LGN, primary visual cortex (V1), visual association cortex, and the vestibular system (Zeki, 1993). When the eyes move, the frontal eye fields (FEF) direct the choice of visual targets through input to the SC and premotor neurons of the brainstem (Farah, 2000; Tong, 2003). The FEF may also suppress eye movements (Culham, Cavanaugh, & Kanwisher, 2001). The right FEF controls leftward horizontal gaze shifts, while the left FEF controls horizontal gaze shifts to the right. With input from the primary visual cortex feeding forward to the superior colliculi we are able to maintain posture, direct our movements, and orient ourselves in space. The cortex and the reticular formation of the brainstem feedback to the LGN creating a sensorimotor feedback loop (Kandel et al., 1995).

In summary, the processing of picture, object, and graphic language stimuli begins at the retina and branches off into distinct but interactive visual networks that serve object identification, action on objects, and directed eye movements. Efficient visual processing involves well-coordinated eye movements, the ability to maintain fixation, and the timely identification, localization, and integration of visual input at the cortical level. In the following pages the reader will learn more about how these visual functions are carried out.

SEPARATE PATHWAYS FOR OBJECT IDENTIFICATION AND ACTION: THE VENTRAL AND DORSAL VISUAL PATHWAYS

As they exit the LGN, neural fibers of the visual system spread out to form the optic radiation (Wolf, 2007) (Figure 1-2). Neurons representing the upper visual field are in the lower (ventral) portion of the optic radiation, while those representing the lower visual field are in the upper portion (Farah, 2000). Within the optic radiation cells of the central visual pathway divide into two groups, one dedicated to form recognition and the other to color (Zeki, 1993). Both color and form pathways synapse in primary visual cortex and visual association cortex in the occipital lobe and end within the inferior temporal cortex (Milner & Goodale, 2006) (Figure 1-4). This is called the *ventral pathway* or *what pathway* because it carries information related to the detail of objects and faces (Ungerleider & Mishkin, 1982; Zihl, 2000a). In relation to reading it is also called the *visual word form system* (Vinckier et al., 2007). The fusiform gyrus in the inner, lower aspect of the temporal lobe is particularly important in the recognition of faces, numbers and letters (Brodmann

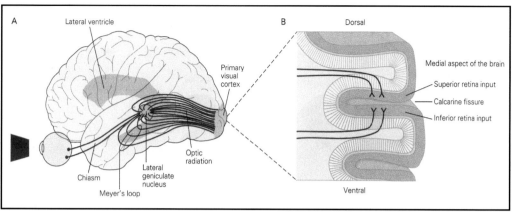

Figure 1-2. The path of visual information from retina to LGN, ending in the primary visual cortex. (A) The early stages of visual processing. Visual processing begins with basic feature analysis and continues to more complex analysis of objects and scenes. Neighboring retinal ganglia send information about motion, color, line orientation, and direction through the optic chiasm and optic tract to the LGN of the thalamus. The LGN regulates, relays, and filters input to and from multiple areas of the cortex including the primary visual cortex and the visual association cortex. The flow of information occurs in both a parallel and sequential manner. (B) A cross-section through the primary visual cortex in the occipital lobe. Fibers that relay input from the inferior half of the retina terminate in the inferior bank of the visual cortex, below the calcarine fissure. Those that relay input from the superior half of the retina terminate in the superior bank. (Reprinted with permission from Kandel, E. R., Schwartz, J. H., & Jessel, T. M. [2000], *Principles of neural science* [4th ed]. New York, NY: McGraw-Hill Education.)

19) (McCandliss, Cohen, & Dehaene, 2003; Pammer et al., 2004; Ramachandran 2004; Wojciulik & Kanwisher, 1999). With regard to reading, Wilson, Rising, Stib, Rapcsak, and Beeson (2013) describe the complex reading process as "a hierarchical posterior-to-anterior gradient of processing in the ventral visual stream, with successive regions coding increasingly larger and more complex perceptual attributes of the letter string."

Information from the peripheral visual system synapses in primary visual cortex and forms the dorsal visual pathway ending within the posterior parietal cortex (Figure 1-4). The ventral stream serves object recognition, while the dorsal stream serves awareness of spatial information (Ungerleider & Mishkin, 1982). For this reason, the dorsal stream is sometimes labeled the *where pathway*. Milner and Goodale (2006) differentiated the perception of attributes of objects (ventral pathway) from the performance of visual motor actions on objects (i.e., the ability to reach toward a target with a specific functional purpose). They proposed that action and perception are separate but interconnected functions of the visual system and relabeled the dorsal pathway as the *how pathway*, because it subconsciously serves visually-guided action. The authors concluded that a functioning visual system depends upon extensive interconnections between these pathways. Koshing et al. (2005) studied interactions between the ventral and dorsal pathways in a mental rotation task and found that the amount of interaction between them increased with the level of complexity and the increase in cognitive load of the assigned task.

The Striate Cortex

The primary visual cortex, also known as *V1*, the *striate cortex* or *calcarine cortex*, is located within the occipital lobes (see Figures 1-1, 1-2). The central 10 degrees of the retina make up 80% of the input to V1, with the remaining 20% from the peripheral retina. Cells within the primary visual cortex code the retinal location for each eye separately and code differences in contrast and orientation (vertical, horizontal) (Kuffler, 1973; Tong, 2003) such as the edges and borders of letters and objects. The majority of the primary visual cortex is concealed within the calcarine fissure and the upper and lower gyri that border it. Retinal input from the lower visual field projects to the upper lip (cuneus) of the calcarine sulcus (CS) (see Figure 1-2). Input from the upper visual field

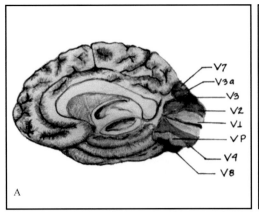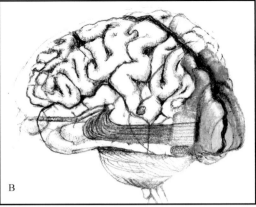

Figure 1-3. Illustration of primary visual cortex and visual association cortex in the occipital lobes. (A) Sagittal view; (B) view of primary visual cortex and visual association cortex. In V1, the neural receptive fields are small. The neurons fire in response to a horizontal line or the edges and borders of letters and objects. In V2 and V4 of the visual cortex, the receptive fields are larger than in V1. The neurons fire in response to more specific objects such as letters and faces.

projects to the lower lip (lingual gyrus) of the CS (Helvie, 2011). Visual input from the peripheral retina projects to the posterior CS at the occipital pole (Zeki, 1993). The horizontal meridian (the imaginary line that separates the upper and lower visual fields) is represented by cells deep within the calcarine sulcus (Fahle, 2003).

The Prestriate Cortex

The area of the occipital lobe anterior to V1 is the prestriate cortex or *association cortex* (Brodmann, 19). This is where visual detail is processed. Divisions of the association cortex are labeled V2, V3, V3a, V4d, V4v, V4C, V8 and so on (see Figure 1-3) (Devinsky and D'Esposito, 2004; Roelfsma, 2006). Together these areas form a narrow band bordering the primary visual cortex in each hemisphere (Ratcliff & Ross, 1981). These labels reflect the segregation of detailed information, the different visual functions these areas undertake (e.g., V3: global motion detection; V5: local motion detection) (Possin, 2010) and their distinct projections within the cortex (Baker, 2000; Tong, 2003). There is a direct correspondence between points on the retina, layers of the LGN, points in V1, and divisions within the visual association cortex. This reflects the retinotopic organization referred to earlier. Elements of form are bound together in the association cortex in a process called *perceptual binding*. The ability to segment or group and then bind features leads to form recognition (Farah, 2000; Wolf, 2007), which is necessary for letter recognition and the activation of letter codes. Interconnections between areas of the visual cortex that represent the center of the visual field present the viewer with an uninterrupted scene as gaze crosses the vertical midline (Hubel, 1995).

The Corpus Callosum

The corpus callosum is a bundle of sensory fibers that integrates the functions of the right and left cortical hemispheres. Information relating to vertical midline is communicated interhemispherically and integrated for motor, somatosensory, and written language systems through the corpus callosum, including binocular information that is necessary for stereopsis (depth perception) (Gazzaniga, 2000; Hubel, 1995; Miller et al., 1999; Saint-Amour, Lepore, Lassonde, & Guillemot, 2004). We know from split-brain studies that damage to the corpus callosum will result in impaired recognition of the printed word, because input to the right hemisphere

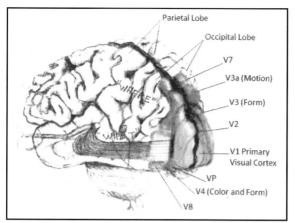

Figure 1-4. The ventral (what) and dorsal (where) visual pathways.

(via the left nasal and right temporal retina) can no longer be transmitted to the left hemisphere through the corpus callosum (Sperry, 1968; Buklina, 2005).

The Cerebellum

The cerebellum is located beneath the occipital lobes and is composed of both gray and white matter. The cerebellum plays a role in the coordinated actions of voluntary muscle movements including those for speech (Highnam & Bleile, 2011; Riecker et al., 2005) and fine visual-motor control (Nakamagoe, Iwamoto, & Yoshida, 2000). The cerebellum interacts with the brainstem to achieve accurate eye position for sustained gaze. It plays a role in initiating and maintaining visual pursuit movements for tracking moving objects (Alexander & Slinger-Constant, 2004; Moschner et al., 1999; Nawrot & Rizzo, 1994). In the remainder of this chapter we will review the motor and sensory components of vision and their role in language and cognition.

THE MOTOR AND SENSORY COMPONENTS OF VISION

The Motor Components of Vision

Voluntary and reflexive eye movements are necessary to perceive and track objects (Gillen, 2009). Information relating to spatial relationships between the viewer and objects (e.g., distance, depth, orientation) and between objects or words is recalibrated with each movement of the eyes (Russell et al., 2010; Sanet & Press, 2011). Five coordinated movements adjust focus for viewing at different distances, shift gaze among stationary objects, and track moving objects. These are: 1) counter-rolling, 2) smooth pursuits, 3) vergence, 4) saccades, and 5) fixation.

The eye movements that allow us to track moving objects or to fixate objects while we are moving are counter-rolling and smooth pursuits. Counter-rolling keeps the eyes fixated on a target when the head moves away from it in any direction. The vestibulo-ocular reflex is responsible for keeping the eyes focused on a target by shifting gaze in the direction opposite head movement (Roeser, Valent, & Hosford-Dunn, 2007). Smooth pursuits are fast, volitional movements associated with finding and following a target. The eyes move together horizontally, vertically, and diagonally in order to track objects and to keep them stable on the central retina where vision is the sharpest (Sanet & Press, 2011).

Focusing for Near Tasks

Reading and writing are acquired skills built upon the foundation of auditory-verbal language acquisition. Unlike speech and audition they require structured training (Brownsett & Wise, 2010; Dehaene, 2009; Magrassi, Bongetta, Bianchini, Berardesca, & Arienta, 2010;). Three eye movements are integrated in the act of focusing for near tasks such as reading and writing (Gentile, 1997): 1) convergence, 2) pupil constriction, and 3) thickening of the lens.

Convergence, or rotation of the eyes toward midline, brings objects that are approaching, and stationary objects at near distances into focus. The pupils constrict, and the lens thickens reflexively. The elastic quality of the lens allows for a sharp image at near and far distances. Pupil constriction impedes visual input from the peripheral visual fields to the cornea and iris, which improves visual clarity for near objects and print. Pupil constriction is mediated by the retinotectal pathway of the midbrain (Hammond, 2000; Kandel et al., 1995). Contraction of the ciliary muscle relaxes the ligaments that suspend the lens causing it to thicken and take on a more spherical shape. Thickening of the lens increases its ability to break up light waves (i.e., refractive power) when we focus on near objects.

Movement of the eyes toward midline or away from midline is called *vergence*. Vergence movements occur when we adjust our distance of focus through accommodation, the ability to shift focus from a distant target to a near target and vice versa. The eyes turn outward (i.e., divergence) when viewing distant objects and move toward midline when viewing near objects (i.e., convergence) (Adler, 1965; Gillen, 2009; Titcomb, Okoye, & Schiff, 1997) (e.g., when looking from the road to the dashboard while driving). As the eyes converge the distance of focus is adjusted through contraction of the ciliary muscle, which is innervated by CN III in the midbrain (Gillen, 2009; Hubel, 1995). For a more detailed description see Ciuffreda et al. (2007).

Reading and writing involve convergence, saccades, and fixations (Brownsett & Wise, 2010; Ciuffreda & Kapoor, 2007). These eye movements are highly correlated with reading efficiency. Convergence keeps the eyes aligned during the repeated fixations and saccadic movements that occur with reading. Saccades are quick eye movements that center the objects of our attention on the fovea, where vision is the sharpest (Martin, 2004; Rayner & Pollatsek, 1987). This is important for letter discrimination (Greenlee, 2003; Schuett, Heywood, Kentridge, & Zihl, 2008b). Microsaccades are fast (.25 milliseconds) small, conjugate (i.e., eyes move together in the same direction), involuntary movements that recenter an image on the fovea during fixation (Rayner, 1998; Reichle, Pollatsek, Fisher, & Rayner, 1998; Tse et al., 2010).

Microsaccades play an important role in object identification and in reading because they renew the image projected to the retina by repeatedly stimulating retinal ganglia to fire during sustained fixation (Engbert & Kliegl, 2003; Hautala & Parviainen, 2014; Martinez-Conde, Macknik, & Hubel, 2004; Martinez-Conde, Macknik, Troncoso, & Dyar, 2006).

Control of the timing and speed of saccades is mediated by the superior colliculi of the midbrain, FEF, dorsolateral prefrontal cortex, posterior parietal cortex, primary visual cortex, and basal ganglia (Farah, 2000; Greenlee, 2003; Tong, 2003). In languages such as English with a left-to-right scan pattern, the reader makes approximately 3 saccades per second (Ross & Ma-Wyatt, 2004; Wang & Pan, 2013). Word shape and length as viewed by the right parafoveal retina determine the length of each new saccade (Leff, Scott, Crewes, Hodgson, & Cowey, 2004).

Fixation and the Perceptual Span

Fixation is the act of maintaining steady and accurate gaze at a visual target (Gillen, 2009). When we read, fixations tend to be located just to the left of the middle of a word, regardless of word length (Rayner, 1979). The ability to identify the first two to three letters is linked to the reader's ability to access the mental lexicon (i.e., orthographic lexicon). Within a single fixation, skilled readers are able to identify three to four letters to the left of the point of fixation and approximately 14 letters or letter spaces to the right of fixation (McConkie & Rayner, 1975). This is the *perceptual span*, also referred to in reading as the *visual span* (Legge et al, 2009). With each successive saccade the perceptual span moves ahead seven to nine letters (Kim & Lemke, 2016; Rayner, 1998). The length of the perceptual span or visual span is normally limited by acuity (Legge et al., 2009). As the length of the perceptual span is greater than a single word, there is overlap in word processing with each successive fixation (Rayner & Bertera, 1979). In silent reading, fixations are reported to last between 200 and 500 milliseconds (Wolf, 2007). The likelihood that a word will be fixated is greater if it has semantic content (i.e., if it can be defined), has grammatical purpose (i.e., function words), and if it is among the longer words in a passage (Rayner & Duffy, 1986; Rayner & McConkie, 1976). Within the perceptual span, letters are processed in parallel for familiar words and are processed serially (i.e., letter-by-letter) for unfamiliar words (Coltheart, Rastle, Perry, Langdon, & Ziegler, 2001; Hautala & Parviainen, 2014).

Information that is detected in the right parafoveal field is used to process text on subsequent fixations. This early processing of words to the right of fixation means there is less processing time needed once a word has been fixated (Rayner, Liversedge, & White, 2006; Rayner, White, Kambe, Miller, & Liversedge, 2003). Early (prelexical) visual processing of text and the perceptual span are influenced by attentional factors mediated by the frontoparietal cortex (Russell, Malhorta, & Husain, 2004; Schuett et al., 2008b). Rayner, Slattery, and Belanger (2010) summarized the findings of several studies of the perceptual span. The authors concluded that children who are just learning to read, people with dyslexia, and older adult readers have a shorter perceptual span than college-level readers. The slower readers in each of these studies found it difficult to process fixated words and this caused them to pay less attention to words in the right parafoveal field (Rayner, 1986; Rayner, Castelhano, & Yang, 2009; Rayner, Murphy, Henderson, & Pollatsek, 1989).

Sensory Components of Vision

The sensory components of vision include the perception of light, color, texture, and contrast and the binding of these elements into visual images. Formal testing of the sensory components of vision includes measures of visual acuity, visual fields, binocular function, contrast sensitivity, form recognition, depth perception, and spatial perception. These tests are performed by an occupational therapist, neurooptometrist, or ophthalmologist.

Visual Acuity

Visual acuity refers to the clarity of spatially separable objects (Leff & Starrfelt, 2014). Measures of visual acuity are reported as 20/x, where x equals the distance in feet at which the individual with normal vision could view an object clearly. 20/20 is normal vision. 20/60 means the viewer sees at 20 feet what a person with normal vision could see at 60 feet. Consult with an occupational therapist or neurooptometrist regarding methods for testing visual acuity for near distances.

Visual Fields

Visual field testing measures the ability to perceive light, color, objects and movement in central vision and in all four quadrants of the visual field. The temporal visual field extends to approximately 90 degrees, while the nasal visual field extends to 60 degrees (Margolis, 2011) (Figure 1-5). Performance on visual field testing reflects function from the level of the retina through the visual pathways to the visual cortex. Visual field testing is highly relevant to reading comprehension, because information detected from the right parafoveal field is used to process text on subsequent fixations (Rayner et al., 2003).

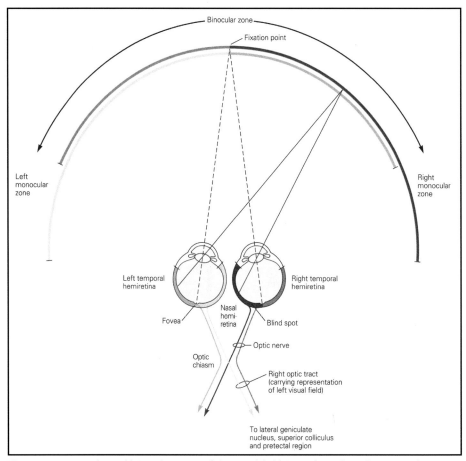

Figure 1-5. Monocular and binocular zones of the visual field. Input from the right monocular zone is projected to the ipsilateral right nasal hemiretina (see dark band delineating right monocular zone) but not to the left. Beyond the optic chiasm, this information is combined with input from the left temporal hemiretina and projected to the left visual cortex. Visual information from the binocular zone provides input to each eye. In this figure, input from the right binocular zone stimulates the right nasal hemiretina as well as the left temporal hemiretina. (Reprinted with permission from Kandel, E. R., Schwartz, J. H., & Jessel, T. M. [2000], *Principles of neural science* [4th ed]. New York, NY: McGraw-Hill Education.)

Crowding

Letter identification is influenced by *crowding*, which is caused when letters that flank a target letter interfere with recognition of the target letter (Legge et al., 2009; Pelli et al., 2004; 2007), and by visual acuity which diminishes with increasing distance from the point of fixation (Schotter et al., 2012). Pelli et al., (2007) define crowding as "…excessive feature integration, inappropriately including extra features that spoil recognition of the target object." Both crowding and visual acuity restrict the length of the peripheral or visual span (the number of words recognized with one fixation) and the ability to identify words in the parafoveal visual field.

Contrast Sensitivity

Contrast sensitivity is the ability to distinguish objects within a scene by detecting differences in light intensity and wavelength. Objects are more easily detected when they contrast more sharply with the background. Two types of retinal ganglia are found among the ganglia of the central and peripheral visual pathways. These cells have a *receptive field center* and a *receptive field surround* that act in opposition to one another (Baker, 2000; Hubel, 1995; Kandel, et al., 1995). They

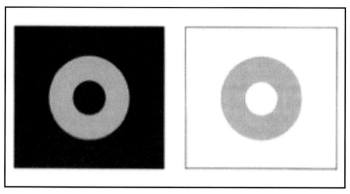

Figure 1-6. The appearance of an object depends principally on the contrast between the object and its background, not on the intensity of the light source. The two gray rings in the figure are identical in hue, but they appear to have different brightness because the different backgrounds produce different contrasts. (Reprinted with permission from Kandel, E. R., Schwartz, J. H., & Jessel, T. M. [2000], *Principles of neural science* [4th ed]. New York, NY: McGraw-Hill Education.)

are called *on-* and *off-center cells.* On-center cells respond to a rapid increase in the intensity of light that strikes the center of the cell's receptive field. When light hits the receptive field surround, the cell's response is inhibited (Figure 1-6; Wolf, 2007). Off-center retinal ganglion cells fire in response to a rapid decrease in light intensity within the center of the cell's receptive field, or when light is applied to the receptive surround. Hubel (1995) explains: "An off-center cell discharges at its highest rate in response to a black spot on a white background, because we are now illuminating only the surround of its receptive field." The overlap of adjacent ganglion cells in the retina causes a single stimulus to be spread to hundreds of other on- and off-center cells (Roelfsema, 2006). This neural response to contrast reveals the borders and edges of forms so that we are able to distinguish individual objects within a scene (Farah, 2000). Contrast sensitivity is a critical component of the reading process because it allows us to see the fine detail of print. This is particularly important as we age (Brussee, van den Berg, van Nisen, & van Rens, 2017).

Spatial Perception

Spatial perception includes the accurate location of horizontal and vertical midline, object constancy (i.e., recognizing objects in different views), size constancy, and a stable representation of object location (i.e., the ability to discriminate eye movements from object movements) (Fahle, 2003). A review of the literature on visual spatial function clarifies the integrated components of spatial perception (Table 1-1) (Possin, 2010). The ventral visual pathway transmits information on object form and color, while the dorsal visual pathway processes input on object movement and location. Visual-spatial cognition involves both subconscious bottom-up processes (i.e., bits of information are bound together into recognizable forms) (Medina et al., 2009; Wolfe & Bennett, 1997) and top-down processes (i.e., integration with previous knowledge and expectations). These bottom-up and top-down processes feed forward and backward to refine our perceptions (Ciuffreda et al., 2007; Fahle, 2003; Han & Lehnerstrand, 1999; Padula, 1996).

Judgements about location and spatial orientation depend upon the viewer's frame of reference (e.g., egocentric/viewer centered vs allocentric/object centered) (Halligan et al., 2003; Marsh & Hillis, 2008; Medina et al., 2009; Milner & Goodale, 2006). When the frame of spatial reference is egocentric, object midline is perceived relative to the center of the viewer's retina, head, or body. When the spatial frame of reference is allocentric the location of one item is defined relative to the location of other items in the scene. In this case, midline perception may be either object- or stimulus-centered. In an *object-centered* frame of reference, the center of an object defines midline, regardless of the object's location across the visual field. However, when objects have a canonical, or typical left-right, spatial orientation such as the left-right orientation of letters in a word, the viewer's frame of reference is *stimulus-centered.* This means that the perceived left and right halves of the object remain constant, regardless of its location or whether the object stands on end or is flipped end for end. This has implications for a discussion of perceptual neglect in Chapter 2 (see Table 2-1).

TABLE 1-1	
COMPONENTS OF VISUAL SPATIAL PROCESSING	
BOTTOM-UP COGNITION	• Detects color, form/shape, and line orientation • Recognizes faces • Right-left orientation • Recognizes whether letters and numbers are facing the correct direction • Detects motion and location information
TOP-DOWN COGNITION	• Selects visual information for detailed processing • Organizes complex visual information • Mediates voluntary shifts of attention • Inhibits irrelevant information • Plans how to use visual information to achieve behavioral goals • Unifies percepts of ambiguous visual stimuli • Manipulates and updates information from bottom-up systems in the posterior cortex
VENTRAL PATHWAY	• Detects non-spatial features that determine object identity such as color and form • Processes input from the contralateral visual field through the corpus callosum
DORSAL PATHWAY	• Detects object location and movement • Relates motor movement to object function
EGOCENTRIC REFERENCE FRAME	• Processes object locations in reference to viewer's own location • Involves caudate nucleus, parietal cortex
ALLOCENTRIC REFERENCE FRAME	• Process object locations relative to the location of other objects, independent of the viewer's location • Involves hippocampus in medial temporal lobe
Adapted from Possin, K. (2010). Visual spatial cognition in neurodegenerative disease. *Neurocase*, 16(6), 466-487.	

DUAL INTEGRATED NETWORKS FOR VISUAL ATTENTION

Current theories of spatial perception, attention, and perceptual neglect have evolved from a focus on site of lesion to a study of the physiological signs associated with neglect. Corbetta and Shulman (2011) and others (Siegel, Donner, Oostenveld, Fries, & Engel, 2008) have reviewed the extensive body of literature on hemispatial neglect and have identified two interactive but distinct networks that modulate attention and awareness:

1. A *dorsal frontoparietal attention network*, involved with spatial functions
2. A *ventral frontoparietal attention network*, involved with nonspatial functions

TABLE 1-2		
DUAL INTEGRATED NETWORKS OF ATTENTION		
	DORSAL FRONTOPARIETAL ATTENTION NETWORK	**VENTRAL FRONTOPARIETAL ATTENTION NETWORK**
CORTICAL LOCATION	• Medial intraparietal sulcus (MIPS) • Superior longitudinal fasciculus (SPL), precuneus • Supplementary eye fields (SEF) • Frontal eye fields (FEF)	• Temporoparietal junction (TPJ) • Inferior parietal lobule/superior temporal gyrus (IPL/STG) • Visual frontal cortex (VFC) • Inferior frontal gyrus/medial frontal gyrus (IFG/MFG)
CORTICAL ORGANIZATION	• Symmetrically organized bilaterally	• Lateralized primarily to the right hemisphere
PHYSIOLOGICAL SIGNALS	• Spatial attention • Eye movement • Saliency • Egocentric frame of reference • Contains maps of contralateral space • Interhemispheric interactions	• Maintains arousal • Maintains vigilance • Reorients to unexpected events

Adapted from Corbetta, M., and Shulman, G. (2011). Spatial neglect and attention networks. *Annual Review of Neuroscience, 34,* 569-599.

The dorsal frontoparietal attention network is symmetrically organized in the right and left hemisphere. Each hemisphere contains a map of contralateral space. The dorsal network acts to disengage attention, control eye movements, and modulate spatial attention in an egocentric frame of reference (Table 1-2). The ventral frontoparietal attention network responds to novel events, reorients to novel stimuli, and maintains arousal and vigilance. It is lateralized primarily to the right hemisphere (Corbetta & Shulman, 2011).

Attention may be overt or covert. Fixated objects (where the image falls on the central retina) receive overt attention that shifts from one object to another through saccadic eye movements. In English and other languages with a left to right scan pattern, covert attention shifts rightward to words that fall outside the central retina at a new location, just before a rightward saccadic shift occurs to that new location (Posner & Petersen, 1990; Rayner, 1998; Sereno, 1992; Schneider & Deubel, 1995).

Silver, Ress, and Heeger (2005) examined the response of the posterior parietal cortex in covert attention tasks. Test subjects were instructed to overtly fixate a central point while covertly attending to stimuli presented at consecutive points around the periphery of the fixation point (e.g., as numbers around a clock face). Two areas within the intraparietal sulcus responded when covert attention was directed to stimuli outside the central point of fixation to stimuli in the contralateral field. These areas were topographically organized. The authors concluded that the parietal cortex is involved in covert attention.

Subcortical structures are also engaged in attention. The superior colliculi of the midbrain shift attention toward new targets and the pulvinar of the thalamus filters out visual stimuli to enhance attention to a new salient target (Corbetta & Shulman, 2011; Posner & Peterson, 1990).

FORM RECOGNITION AND READING

Form and color vision are mediated by the ventral (central) visual pathway. Lines and shapes of different directional orientation (e.g. \ / l) are bound into recognizable forms. This ability begins within the first year of life with gradual recognition of objects based on the convergence of edges that form T, Y, or L shapes (Dehaene, 2009; Dehaene & Cohen, 2011). At the earliest stages, objects, words, or facial features are detected without conscious awareness (Fahle, 2003; Wolf, 2007). Wolfe and Bennett (1997) describe perception at this early stage as "shapeless bundles of basic features." When we read and write, form perception differentiates similar letters (e.g., b/q, b/d) and words (e.g., pop/pod) andidentifieswordboundarieswithinasentence. Form recognition is a peripheral, or bottom-up component of reading.

Visual word forms are strings of letters that are perceived as invariant, regardless of differences in color, font, size of characters, visual field location, etc. A number of studies have identified a visual word form area (VWFA) or *letter-box area* in the occipitotemporal sulcus at the border of the left fusiform gyrus (Cohen et al., 2000; Cohen & Dehaene, 2004; Cohen et al., 2003; Molko et al., 2002; Starrfelt, Habekost, & Leff, 2009; Warrington & Shallice, 1980). This area contains cells that are important in the recognition of faces, numbers, letters, and words (McCandliss et al., 2003; Pammer et al., 2004; Ramachandran, 2004). Tarkiainen, Helenius, Hansen, Cornelissen, and Salmelin (1999) and Tarkiainen, Cornelius, and Salmelin (2002) studied the brain's response to words and faces using magnetoencephalography. The authors found that cells were activated within 100 milliseconds (msecs) of fixation. After another 50 msecs the VWFA in the left hemisphere was activated in response to words, while the homologous area of the right hemisphere activated in response to faces. McCandliss et al. (2003) have theorized that the VWFA "… mediates between specific (visual) input, and more abstract linguistic areas responsible for lexical, semantic and phonological processes." These processes are engaged in reading and spelling. Rapid recognition of letters and words is important for efficient comprehension and recall of reading material (Flowers et al., 2004). Wolf (2007) states, "If we recognize symbols at almost automatic speeds, we can allocate more time to mental processes that are continuously expanding when we read and write." The author concludes: "The efficient reading brain … quite literally has more time to think." A frequent complaint of neurologically impaired clients is that they cannot remember what they read. The potential impact of slow processing on reading comprehension and memory for graphic material is nicely illustrated in Wolf's (2007) timeline of reading.

DUAL ROUTE MODEL OF READING AND WRITING

The dual route model of reading and writing proposes that the production of written words occurs through a phonological route relying on phoneme-grapheme conversion, or through a lexical route that provides direct access to long-term memory storage for all known words (i.e., the orthographic lexicon) (Purcell, Turkeltaub, Eden, & Rapp, 2011; Rapcsak, Henry, Teague, Carnahan, & Beeson, 2007; Rodrigues, Fontoura, & de Salles, 2014). Research in the field of cognitive neuropsychology supports this theory (Hillis, 2001). Early learners need a strong foundation in phonology (i.e., how sounds are combined to make words) in order to learn to read and write. In addition to phonological awareness, reading acquisition is dependent upon rapid naming ability and perhaps even higher-level executive skills, including the ability to retrieve, retain, and manipulate information as it is processed (Alexander & Slinger-Constant, 2004; Baddeley, 2012).

Computer models of reading have demonstrated that for at-risk young readers, learning is most efficient when the orthographic-semantic (i.e., sight word) pathway and the orthographic-phono-logic (i.e., letter-sound) pathway work together to decode words (Alexander & Slinger-Constant, 2004; Harm & Seidenberg, 1999).

Peripheral Components of Writing

Like reading, writing and spelling involve formal training (Dehaene, 2009) and like speech acquisition, writing and typing are dependent on visual-motor coordination, visual-perceptual skills, and somatosensory feedback (Brownsett & Wise, 2010). Writing and spelling engage both central and peripheral processes through a network of cortical and subcortical regions (Planton, Jucla, Roux, & Demonet, 2013). The central components of writing include the retrieval, selection, and sequencing of letters and words from long-term memory (i.e., orthographic lexicon) according to phonological (grapheme-to-phoneme conversion), lexical (phoneme-to-grapheme conversion), and semantic rules (Dufor & Rapp, 2013; Purcell, 2011; Rapcsak & Beeson, 2002).

Allographic processing is a key component of writing. Abstract letter identities are coded or transformed into *allographs* by assigning letter names and graphic features (e.g., capital or lower case; print or cursive, single or doubled letters [e.g. lesson], syllable structure, CV status) (Caramazza & Micelli, 1990; Buchwald & Rapp 2006; Jonsdottir, Shallice, & Wise, 1996; Lambert et al., 2007). Allographs are drawn in a particular sequence and arrangement of strokes accord-ing to learned motor plans (Buchwald & Rapp, 2009; Jonsdottir et al., 1996; Menichelli, Rapp, & Semenza, 2008; Purcell et al., 2011; Rapcsak & Beeson, 2002). The peripheral, motor components of writing involve grasping and hand placement functions (Castiello, 2005), as well as the plan-ning and execution of learned motor sequences (Dufor & Rapp, 2013; van Galen, 1991). As hand movements follow eye movements, written letter formation, sequencing, and spacing depend upon accurate saccadic eye movements and intact spatial perception (Land, 2006; Purcell et al., 2011). In a meta-analysis of 18 imaging studies of writing, including mental writing, finger writing in the air, typewriting, and writing with pen on paper (with and without visual guidance), Planton and colleagues (2013) found the most frequent area of activation was in Brodmann area 6 in the left premotor cortex, which includes a portion of the FEF. The reader will recall that the FEF are involved in the control of saccadic eye movements (Farah, 2000; Tong, 2003). Functional magnetic resonance imaging studies of letter writing and written spelling also show activation of the VWFA (Dufor & Rapp, 2013). As noted previously, this area plays a perceptual role within the ventral visual pathway and is associated with recognition of invariant letter and word forms in reading print and script (Molko et al., 2002; Qaio et al., 2010).

Working Memory in Oral and Written Spelling

Over the past four decades, oral and written spelling have been studied extensively in adults with and without acquired brain injury. It has been repeatedly demonstrated that both types of spelling engage long-term and working memory processes (Buchwald & Rapp, 2006, 2009). This is important to the rehabilitation of acquired reading and writing disorders (see Chapter 3). Baddeley and Hitch (1974) proposed a model of working memory as a system of multiple components that support temporary information storage for the performance of complex cognitive functions (see also Baddeley, 1996, 2000, 2012). This model has three components: the central executive for atten-tional control and two subsystems that serve this central executive: a *phonological loop* (or *pho-nological buffer*) that has both storage and rehearsal functions, and a *visuospatial sketchpad* (also called the *graphemic buffer* or *orthographic buffer*). According to the Baddeley model, memory decay is avoided through subvocalization, or rehearsal, of letter names or sequences of items. This forms a memory trace in the phonological buffer. The visuospatial sketchpad acts as a working memory component for writing and typing. Words are retrieved from long-term memory and held briefly in the visuospatial sketchpad until they are converted to letter names (in oral spelling) and graphemes (in writing) (Menichelli et al., 2012; Purcell, Napoliello, & Eden, 2011a). This theory is supported by a number of studies of reading (Buchwald & Rapp, 2009; Jonsdottir et al., 1996; Kan et al., 2006).

Several studies have demonstrated that the primary function of the phonological loop is to act as a temporary memory store for new words in early language acquisition, in developmentally later acquisition of more abstract words, and in learning the unfamiliar phonologic sequences of a foreign language. Working memory ability is associated with reading skill and with the accuracy, efficiency, and speed of phonological processing. This has been demonstrated for younger readers and adults, individuals with specific language impairment, and in polyglots (Brady, 1986; Daneman and Carpenter, 1980). Baddeley, Gathercole, and Papagno (1998) proposed that the phonological loop supports the acquisition of syntax because it facilitates "learning a storehouse of multiword language patterns that are used both as models for his or her own utterances and for the abstraction of the rules governing connected language." In Chapter 2 we will explore the relationship of the motor and sensory components of vision to language and cognition, and review how these processes are vulnerable to aging, acquired brain stroke, trauma, and progressive neurological disease.

REFERENCES

Adler, F. H. (1965). Ocular motility. In: *Physiology of the eye: Clinical application*. St. Louis, MO: C. V. Mosby.

Alexander, A.W. & Slinger-Constant, A-M. (2004). Current status of treatments for dyslexia: Critical review. *Journal of Child Neurology, 19*(10), 744-758.

Baddeley, A. D. (1996). The fractionation of working memory. Colloquium Paper, *Proceedings of the National Academy of Sciences, 93,* 13468-13472.

Baddeley, A. D. (2000). The episodic buffer: A new component of working memory? *Trends in Cognitive Science, 4*(11), 412-423.

Baddeley, A. D. (2012). Working memory: Theories, models and controversies. *Annual Review of Psychology, 63,* 1-29.

Baddeley, A. D. & Hitch, G. J. (1974). Working memory. *Psychology of Learning and Motivation, 8,* 47-89.

Baddeley, A. D., Gathercole, S.E., & Papagno, C. (1998). The phonological loop as a language learning device. *Psychological Review, 105,* 158-173.

Baker, G. E. (2000). Visual pathways, module 2, parts 1 & 3. *Optometry Today.*

Brady, S. (1986). Short-term memory, phonological processing, and reading ability. *Annals of Dyslexia, 36,* 138-153.

Brownsett, S. L. & Wise, R. J. (2010). The contribution of the parietal lobes to speaking and writing. *Cerebral Cortex, 20*(3), 517-523.

Brussee, T., van den Berg, T. J., van Nisen, R. M., & van Rens, G. H. (2017). Associations between spatial and temporal contrast sensitivity and reading. *Optometry and Vision Science, 94*(3), 329-338.

Buchwald, A. & Rapp, B. (2006). Consonants and vowels in orthographic representations. *Cognitive Neuropsychology, 23*(2), 308-337.

Buchwald, A. & Rapp, B. (2009). Distinctions between orthographic long-term memory and working memory. *Cognitive Neuropsychology, 26*(8), 724-751.

Buklina, S. B. (2005). The corpus callosum, interhemispheric interactions, and the function of the right hemisphere of the brain. *Neuroscience and Behavioral Psychology, 35*(5), 473-480.

Buonomano, D.V. & Merzenich, M. M. (1998). Cortical plasticity: From synapses to maps. *Annual Reviews Neuroscience, 21,* 149-186.

Caramazza, A. & Micelli, G. (1990). The structure of orthographic representations in spelling. *Cognition, 37,* 243-297.

Castiello, U. (2005). The neuroscience of grasping. *Nature Reviews Neuroscience, 6,* 726-736.

Ciuffreda, K. J. & Kapoor, N. (2007). Oculomotor dysfunctions, their remediation, and reading-related problems in mild traumatic brain injury. *Journal of Behavioral Optometry, 18*(3), 72-77.

Ciuffreda, K. J., Kapoor, N., Rutner, D., Suchoff, I. B., Han, M. E., & Craig, S. (2007). Occurrence of oculomotor dysfunction in acquired brain injury: A retrospective analysis. *Optometry, 78,* 155-161.

Cohen, L. & Dehaene, S. (2004). Specialization within the ventral stream: The case for the visual word form area. *Neuroimage, 22*(1), 466-476.

Cohen, L., Martinaud, O., Lemer, C., Lehericy, S., Samson, Y., Obadia, M., ... Dehaene, S. (2003). Visual word recognition in the left and right hemispheres: Anatomical and functional correlates of peripheral alexias. *Cerebral Cortex, 13,* 1313-1333.

Cohen, L., Dehaene, S., Naccace, L., Lehericy, S., Dehaene-Lambertz, G., Henaff, M-A., & Michel F. (2000). The visual word form area. *Brain, 123*(2), 291-307.

Coltheart, M., Rastle, K., Perry, C., Langdon, R., & Ziegler, J. (2001). DRC: A dual route cascaded model of visual word recognition and reading aloud. *Psychological Reviews, 108*, 204-256.

Corbetta, M. & Shulman, G. (2011). Spatial neglect and attention networks. *Annual Review of Neuroscience, 34*, 569-599.

Culham, J., Cavanaugh, P., & Kanwisher, N. (2001). Attention response functions: Characterizing brain areas using fMRI activation during parametric variations of attentional load. *Neuron, 32*, 737-746.

Daneman, M. & Carpenter, P. (1980). Individual differences in working memory and reading. *Journal of Verbal Learning and Verbal Behavior, 19*, 450-466.

de Gelder, B. (2010). Uncanny sight in the blind. *Scientific American, 302*(5), 60-65.

Dehaene, S. (2009). *Reading in the Brain: The science and evolution of a human invention.* New York, NY: Viking Books.

Dehaene, S. & Cohen, L. (2011). The unique role of the visual word form area in reading. *Trends in Cognitive Sciences, 15*(6), 254-262.

Devinsky, O. & D'Esposito, M. (2004). *Neurology of cognitive and behavioral disorders.* New York, NY: Oxford University Press.

Diederich, N. J., Stebbins, G., Schlitz, C., & Goetz, C.G. (2014). Are patients with Parkinson's disease blind to blindsight? *Brain, 137*(6), 1838-1849.

Dijkerman, H. C., Milner, D., & Carey, D. P. (1998). Grasping spatial relationships: Failure to demonstrate allocentric visual coding in a patient with visual form agnosia. *Consciousness and Cognition, 7*(3), 424-437.

Dufor, O. & Rapp, B. (2013). Letter representations in writing: An fMRI adaptation approach. *Frontiers in Psychology, 4*, 1-14.

Dutton, G. N. (2003). Cognitive vision, its disorders and differential diagnosis in adults and children: Knowing where and what things are. *Eye, 17*, 289-304.

Engbert, R. & Kliegl, R. (2003). Microsaccades uncover the orientation of covert attention. *Vision Research, 43*, 1035-1045.

Fahle, M. (2003). Failures of visual analysis: Scotoma, agnosia and neglect. In: M. Fahle, & M. Greenlee (Eds.), *The Neuropsychology of Vision* (pp. 179-258). New York, NY: Oxford University Press.

Farah, M. J. (2000). *The cognitive neuroscience of vision.* Malden, MA: Blackwell Publishing.

Flowers, D.L., Jones, K., Noble, K., VanMeter, J., Zeffiro, T. A., Wood, F. B., & Eden, G. F. (2004). Attention to single letters activates left extrastriate cortex. *Neuroimage, 21*, 829-839.

Gazzaniga, M.S. (2000). Cerebral specialization and interhemispheric communication: Does the corpus callosum enable the human condition? *Brain, 123*, 1293-1326.

Gentile, M. (Ed.) (1997). *Functional visual behavior: A therapist's guide to evaluation and treatment options.* Bethesda, MD: American Occupational Therapy Association, Inc.

Gillen, G. (2009). *Cognitive and perceptual rehabilitation: Optimizing function.* St. Louis, MO: Mosby Elsevier.

Grainger, J. & Holcomb, P.J. (2009). Watching the word go by: On the time-course of component processes in visual word recognition. *Language and Linguistics Compass, 3*(1), 128-156.

Greenlee, M. (2003). Functional magnetic resonance imaging and positron emission tomography studies of motion perception, eye movements and reading. In: M., Fahle & M., Greenlee (Eds.), *The Neuropsychology of Vision.* New York, NY: Oxford University Press.

Halligan, P. W., Fink, G. R., Marshall, J. C. & Vallar, G. (2003). Spatial cognition: Evidence from visual neglect. *Trends in Cognitive Neuroscience, 7*(3), 125-133.

Hammond, C. (2000). *The visual pathways: Disorders of the optic chiasm and beyond.* Optometry Today, City University, London. Module 2, Part 9, 33-37.

Han, Y. & Lehnerstrand, G. (1999). Changes of visual localization induced by eye and neck muscle vibration in normal and strabismic subjects. *Graefe's Archive for Clinical and Experimental Ophthalmology, 237*(10), 815-823.

Harm, M. W. & Seidenberg, M. S. (1999). Phonology, reading acquisition and dyslexia: Insights from connectionist models. *Psychological Review, 106*, 491-528.

Hautala, J. & Parviainen, T. (2014). Gaze position reveals impaired attentional shift during visual word recognition in dysfluent readers. *PLoS ONE, 9*(9), e108937.

Helvie, R. (2011). Neural substrates of vision. In: P. S., Suter, & L. H. Harvey (Eds.), *Vision Rehabilitation: Multidisciplinary Care of the Patient Following Brain Injury* (pp. 45-76). Boca Raton, FL: CRC Press.

Highnam, C. L. & Bleile, K. M. (2011). Language in the cerebellum. *American Journal of Speech-Language Pathology, 20*, 337-347.

Hillis, A. E. (2001). The organization of the lexical system. In: B. Rapp (Ed.). *The Handbook of Cognitive Neuropsychology: What Deficits Reveal About the Human Mind* (pp. 185-210). Philadelphia, PA: Psychology Press.

Hubel, D. H. (1995). The eye. In: *Eye, Brain and Vision* (pp. 33-57). New York, NY: W.H. Freeman and Company.

Jonsdottir, M. K., Shallice, T., & Wise, R. (1996). Phonological mediation and the disorder in spelling: cross-language differences? *Cognition, 59*, 169-197.

Kan, I. P., Biran, I., Thompson-Schill, S. L., & Chatterjee, A. (2006). Letter selection and letter assembly in acquired dysgraphia. *Cognitive Behavioral Neurology, 19*(4), 225-236.

Kandel, E. R., Schwartz, J. H., & Jessel, T. M. (1995). Visual processing by the retina. In: *Essentials of neural science and behavior* (pp. 407-424). East Norwalk, CT: Appleton Lange.

Kandel, E. R. (2006). Simple and complex neuronal systems. In: *In search of memory: The emergence of a new science of mind* (pp. 103-115). New York, NY: W.W. Norton Company, Inc.

Kelly, C., Foxe J., & Garavan, H. (2006). Patterns of normal human brain plasticity after practice and their implications for neurorehabilitation. *Archives of Physical Medicine and Rehabilitation, 87*(12 Suppl. 2), 20-29.

Kim, E. S. & Lemke, S. F. (2016). Behavioural and eye-movement outcomes in response to text-based reading treatment for acquired alexia. *Neuropsychological Rehabilitation, 26*(1), 60-86.

Lambert, J., Giffard, B., Nore, F., de la Sayette, V., Pasquier, F., & Eustache, F. (2007). Central and peripheral agraphia in Alzheimer's disease: from the case of Augustus D to a cognitive neuropsychology approach. *Cortex, 43*(7), 935-951.

Land, M. F. (2006). Eye movements and the control of actions in everyday life. *Progress in Retinal and Eye Research, 25*, 296-324.

Leff, A. & Starrfelt, R. (2014). *Alexia: Diagnosis, treatment and theory.* London, UK: Springer.

Leff, A. P., Scott, S. K., Crewes, H., Hodgson, T. L., & Cowey, D. (2004). Impaired reading in patients with right hemianopia. *Annals of Neurology, 47*, 171-178.

Legge, G.E., Cheung, S.-H., Yu, D., Chung, S.T., Lee, H.-W., & Owens D.P. (2009). The case for the visual span as a sensory bottleneck in reading. *Journal of Vision, 7*(2):9.1-915, 1-25.

Ludlow, C., Hoit, J., Kent, R., Ramig, L., Shrivastav, R., Strand, E., … Sapienza, C. (2008). Translating principles of neural plasticity into research on speech motor control recovery and rehabilitation. *Journal of Speech-Language-Hearing Research, 51*(Suppl. 1), S240-S258.

Magrassi, L., Bongetta, D., Bianchini, S., Berardesca, M., & Arienta, C. (2010). Central and peripheral components of writing critically depend on a defined area of the dominant superior parietal gyrus. *Brain Research, 134*, 145-154.

Margolis, N. W. (2011). Evaluation and treatment of visual field loss and visual-spatial neglect. In: P.S. Suter and L. H. Harvey (Eds.), *Vision rehabilitation: Multidisciplinary care of the patient following brain injury* (pp. 153-192). Boca Raton, FL: CRC Press.

Marsh, F. & Hillis, A. (2008). Dissociation between egocentric and allocentric visuospatial and tactile neglect in acute stroke. *Cortex, 44*, 1215-1220.

Martinez-Conde, S., Macknik, S. L., & Hubel, D. H. (2004). The role of fixational eye movements in visual perception. *Nature Reviews: Neuroscience, 5*, 229-240.

Martinez-Conde, S., Macknik, S. L., Troncoso, X. G., & Dyar, T. (2006). Microsaccades counteract visual fading during fixation. *Neuron, 49*(2), 297-305.

McCandliss, B. D., Cohen, L., & Dehaene, S. (2003). The visual word form area: Expertise for reading in the fusiform gyrus. *Trends in Cognitive Neuroscience, 7*(7), 293-299.

McConkie, G. W. & Rayner, K. (1975). The span of the effective stimulus during a fixation in reading. *Perception Psychophysics, 17*, 578-586.

Medina, J., Kannan, V., Pawlak, M. A., Kleinman, J. T., Newhart, M., Davis, C., … Hillis, A. (2009). Neural substrates of visuospatial processing in distinct reference frames: Evidence from unilateral spatial neglect. *Journal of Cognitive Neuroscience, 21*(11), 2073-2084.

Menichelli, A., Rapp, B., & Semenza, C. (2008). Allographic agraphia: A case study. *Cortex, 44*, 861-868.

Menichelli, A., Machetta, F., Zadini, A., & Semenza, C. (2012). Allograpic agraphia for single letters. *Behavioural Neurology, 25*, 1-12.

Mesulam, M. (1998). From sensation to cognition. *Brain, 121*, 1013-1052.

Miller, L. J., Mittenberg, W., Carey, V. M., McMorrow, M. A., Kashner, T. E., & Weinstein, J. M. (1999). Astereopsis caused by traumatic brain injury. *Archives of Clinical Neuropsychology, 14*(6), 537-543.

Milner, A. D. & Goodale, M. A. (2006). *The visual brain in action* (2nd ed.). New York, NY: Oxford University Press.

Molko, N., Cohen, L., Mangin, J., Chochon, F., Lehericy, S., Le Bihan, D., & Dehaene, S. (2002). Visualizing the neural bases of a disconnection syndrome with diffusion tensor imaging. *Journal of Cognitive Neuroscience, 14*(4), 629-636.

Moschner, C., Crawford, T., Heide, W., Trillenberg, P., Kompf, D., & Kennard, C. (1999). Deficits of smooth pursuit initiation in patients with degenerative cerebellar lesions. *Brain, 122*(11), 2147-2158.

Nakamagoe, K., Iwamoto, Y., & Yoshida, K. (2000). Evidence for brainstem structures participating in oculomotor integration. *Science, 288*(5647), 857-859.

Nawrot, N. & Rizzo, M. (1994). Motion perception deficits from midline cerebellar lesions in human. *Vision Research, 35*(5), 723-731.

Okoye, R. (1997). Neuromotor prerequisites of functional vision. In: M. Gentile (Ed.), *Functional visual behavior: A therapist's guide to evaluation and treatment options.* Bethesda, MD: The American Occupational Therapy Association.

Padula, W. V. (1996). Vision: The Process. In: W. V. Padula (Ed.), *Neuro-Optometric Rehabilitation* (pp. 1-14). Santa Ana, CA: Optometric Extension Program.

Pammer, K., Hansen, P. C., Kringelbach, M. L., Holliday, I., Barnes, G., Hillebrand, A., .. Cornelissen, P. L. (2004). Visual word recognition: The first half second. *Neuroimage, 22*, 1819-1825.

Pelli, D.G., Palomares, M., and Majaj, N.J. (2004). Crowding is unlike ordinary masking: Distinguishing feature integration from detection. *Journal of Vision, 4*, 1136-1169.

Pelli, D.G., Tillman, K.A., Freeman, J., Su, M., Berger, T.D. & Majaj, N.J. (2007). Crowding and eccentricity determine reading rate. *Journal of Vision, 7*(2)20, 1-36.

Planton, S., Jucla, M., Roux, F-E., & Demonet, J-F. (2013). The "handwriting brain": A meta-analysis of neuroimaging studies of motor versus orthographic processes. *Cortex, 49*, 2772-2787.

Posner, M. & Petersen, S. (1990). The attention system of the human brain. *Annual Review of Neuroscience, 13*, 28-42.

Possin, K. (2010). Visual spatial cognition in neurodegenerative disease. *Neurocase, 16*(6), 466-487.

Purcell, J. J., Turkeltaub, P. E., Eden, G. F., & Rapp, B. (2011). Examining the central and peripheral processes of written word production through meta-analysis. *Frontiers of Psychology, 2*, 1-16.

Purcell, J. J., Napoliello, E. M., & Eden, G. F. (2011a). A combined fMRI study of typed spelling and reading. *NeuroImage, 55*, 750-762.

Qaio, E., Vinckier, F., Szwed, M., Naccache, L., Valabregue, R., Dehaene, S., & Cohen, L. (2010). Unconsciously deciphering handwriting: Subliminal invariance for handwritten words in the visual word form area. *NeuroImage, 49*, 1786-1799.

Ramachandran, V. S. (2004). A Brief Tour of Human Consciousness. New York, NY: Pearson Education, Inc.

Rapcsak, S. Z. & Beeson, P. M. (2002). Neuroanatomical correlates of spelling and writing. In: A. R. Hillis (Ed.). *The handbook of adult language disorders: Integrating cognitive neuropsychology, neurology and rehabilitation* (pp. 24-37). New York, NY: Psychology Press.

Rapcsak, S. Z., Henry, M. L., Teague, S. L., Carnahan, S. D., & Beeson, P. M. (2007). Do dual-route models accurately predict reading and spelling performance in individuals with acquired alexia and agraphia? *Neuropsychologia, 45*(11), 2519-2524.

Ratcliff, G. & Ross, J. E. (1981). Visual perception and perceptual disorder. *British Medical Journal, 17*(2), 181-186.

Rayner, K. (1979). Eye guidance in reading: Fixation locations within words. *Perception, 8*(1), 21-30.

Rayner, K. (1986). Eye movements and the perceptual span in beginning and skilled readers. *Journal of Experimental Child Psychology, 41*, 211-236.

Rayner, K. (1998). Eye movements in reading and information processing: 20 years of research. *Psychological Bulletin, 124*, 372-422.

Rayner, K. & Bertera, J. H. (1979). Reading without a fovea. *Science, 206*, 468-469.

Rayner, K. & Duffy, S. (1986). Lexical complexity and fixation times in reading: Effects of word frequency, verb complexity, and lexical ambiguity. *Memory and Cognition, 14*, 191-201.

Rayner, K., Castelhano, M., & Yang, J. (2009). Eye movements and the perceptual span in older and younger readers. *Psychology and Aging, 24*(3), 755-760.

Rayner, K. & McConkie, G.W. (1976). What guides a reader's eye movements? *Vision Research 16*, 829-837.

Rayner, K. & Pollatsek, A. (1987). Eye movements in reading: A tutorial review. In: M. Coltheart (Ed.). *Attention and performance XII: The psychology of reading* (pp. 327-362). London, UK: Erlbaum.

Rayner, K., Murphy, L. A., Henderson, J. M., & Pollatsek, A. (1989). Selective attentional dyslexia. *Cognitive Neuropsychology, 6*, 357-378.

Rayner, K., White, S. J, Kambe, G., Miller, B., & Liversedge, S. P. (2003). On the processing of meaning from parafoveal vision during eye fixations in reading. In: J. Hyönä, R. Radach, & H. Deubel (Eds.). *The mind's eye: Cognitive and applied aspects of eye movement research*. Amsterdam, Netherlands: Elsevier.

Rayner, K., Liversedge, S. P., & White, S. J. (2006). Eye movements when reading disappearing text: The importance of the word to the right of fixation. *Vision Research, 46*, 310-323.

Rayner, K., Slattery, T. J., & Belanger, N. N. (2010). Eye movements, the perceptual span and reading speed. *Psychonomic Bulletin and Review, 17*(6), 834-839.

Reichle, E. D., Pollatsek, A., Fisher, D. L., & Rayner, K. (1998). Toward a model of eye movement control in reading. *Psychological Review, 105*(1), 125-127.

Reinhart, S., Schindler, I., & Kerkhoff G. (2011). Optokinetic stimulation affects word omissions but not stimulus-centered reading errors in paragraph reading in neglect dyslexia. *Neuropsychologia, 49*, 2728-2735.

Riecker, A., Mathiak, K., Wildruber, D., Erb, M., Hertrich, I., Grodd W., & Ackerman, H. (2005). fMRI reveals two distinct cerebral networks subserving speech motor control. *Neurology, 64*(4), 700-706.

Ro, T., & Rafal, R. (2006). Visual restoration in cortical blindness: Insights from natural and TMS-induced blindsight. *Neuropsychological Rehabilitation, 16*(4), 377-396.

Rodrigues, J. C., Fontoura, D. R., & de Salles, J. F. (2014). Acquired dysgraphia in adults following right or left hemisphere stroke. *Dementia & Neuropsychology, 8*(3), 236-242.

Roelfsema, P. R. (2006). Cortical algorithms for perceptual grouping. *Annual Review of Neuroscience, 29*, 203-227.

Roeser, R. J., Valent, M., & Hosford-Dunn, H. (2007). *Audiology Diagnosis* (2nd Ed.). New York, NY: Thieme Medical Publishers, Inc.

Ross, J. & Ma-Wyatt, A. (2004). Saccades actively maintain perceptual continuity. *Nature Neuroscience, 7*(11), 65-69.

Russell, C., Malhotra, P., & Husain, M. (2004). Attention modulates the visual field in healthy observers and parietal patients. *Neuroreport, 15*, 2189-2193.

Russell, C., Deidda, C., Malhotra, P., Crinion, J., Merola, S., & Husain, M. (2010). A deficit of spatial remapping in constructional apraxia after right-hemisphere stroke. *Brain, 133*, 1239-1251.

Saint-Amour, D., Lepore, F., Lassonde, M., & Guillemot, J. P. (2004). Effective binocular integration at the midline requires the corpus callosum. *Neuropsychologia, 42*(2), 164-174.

Sanet, R. B. & Press, L. J. (2011). Spatial vision. In: P. S. Suter, & P. H. Harvey (Eds.), *Vision rehabilitation: Multidisciplinary care of the patient following brain injury* (pp. 77-151). Boca Raton, FL: CRC Press.

Schiff, S. (1997). Anatomy and function of the eye. In: M. Gentile (Ed.). *Functional Visual Behavior: A therapist's guide to evaluation and treatment options.* Bethesda, MD: American Occupational Therapy Association, Inc.

Schneider, W. X. & Deubel, H. (1995). Visual attention and saccadic eye movements: Evidence for obligatory and selective spatial coupling. In: J. M. Findlay, R. Walker, & R. W. Kentridge (Eds.), *Eye movement research: Mechanisms, processes and applications* (pp. 317-324). New York, NY Elsevier Science.

Schneider, K. A., Richter, M. C., & Kastner, S. (2004). Retinotopic organization and functional subdivisions of the human lateral geniculate nucleus: A high-resolution functional magnetic resonance imaging study. *Journal of Neuroscience, 24*(41), 8975-8985.

Schotter, E.R., Angele, B., & Rayner, K. (2012). Parafoveal processing in reading. *Attention, Perception and Psychophysics, 75*: 5-35.

Schuett, S., Heywood, C. A., Kentridge, R. W., & Zihl, J. (2008b). The significance of visual information processing in reading: Insights from hemianopic dyslexia. *Neuropsychologia, 46*, 2495-2462.

Sereno, A. (1992). Programming saccades: The role of attention. In: K. Rayner (Ed.), *Eye movements and visual cognition* (pp. 89-107). New York, NY: Springer-Verlag.

Siegel, M., Donner, T. H., Oostenveld, R., Fries, P., & Engel, A. K. (2008). Neuronal synchronization along the dorsal visual pathway reflects the focus of spatial attention. *Neuron, 60*, 709-719.

Silver, M. A., Ress, D., & Heeger, D. (2005). Topographical maps of visual spatial attention in human parietal cortex. *Journal of Neurophysiology, 94*(2), 1358-1371.

Sperry, R. (1968). Hemisphere deconnection and unity in conscious awareness. *American Psychologist, 23*, 723-733.

Starrfelt, R., Habekost, T., & Leff, A.P. (2009). Too little, too late: Reduced visual span and speech characterize pure alexia. *Cerebral Cortex, 19*, 2880-2890.

Tarkiainen, A., Helenius P., Hansen, P. C., Cornelissen, P. L., & Salmelin, R. (1999). Dynamics of letter string perception in the human occipitotemporal cortex. *Brain, 122*, 2119-2132.

Tarkiainen, A., Cornelius, P. L., & Salmelin, R. (2002). Dynamics of visual feature analysis and object- level processing in face vs. letter-string perception. *Brain, 125*(5), 1125-1136.

Titcomb, R. E., Okoye, R., & Schiff, S. (1997). Introduction to the dynamic process of vision. In: M. Gentile (Ed.), *Functional Visual Behavior: A therapist's guide to evaluation and treatment options* (pp.). Bethesda, MD: American Occupational Therapy Association, Inc.

Tong, R. (2003). Primary visual cortex and visual awareness. *Nature Review Neuroscience, 4*(3), 219-229.

Tse, P., Baumgartner, F., & Greenlee, M. (2010). Event-related functional MRI of cortical activity evoked by microsaccades, small visually-guided saccades, and eyeblinks in human visual cortex. *Neuroimage, 49*(1), 805-816.

Ungerleider, L. G. & Mishkin, M. (1982). Two cortical visual systems. In: D.J. Ingle (Ed.), *Analysis of Visual Behavior* (pp. 549-586). Cambridge, MA: MIT Press.

Van Galen, G.P. (1991). Handwriting: Issues for a psychomotor theory. *Human Movement Science, 10*(2-3), 165-191.

Vinckier, F., Dehaene, S., Jobert, A., Dubus, J. P., Sigman, M., & Cohen, L. (2007). Hierarchical coding of letter strings in the ventral stream: dissecting the inner organization of the visual word-form system. *Neuron, 55*, 143-156.

Wang, J. & Pan, Y. (2013). Eye proprioception may provide real time eye position information. *Neurological Sciences, 34*, 281-286.

Warrington, E. K. & Shallice, T. (1980). Word-form dyslexia. *Brain, 103*, 99-112.

Webb, W. G. & Adler, R. K. (2007). Neurosensory organization of Speech and Hearing. In: R. J. Love, & W. G. Webb (Eds.), *Neurology for the Speech-Language Pathologist* (5th ed., pp. 105-123) St. Louis, MO: Mosby Elsevier.

Whitney, C. & Lavador, M. (2004). Why word length only matters in the left visual field. *Neuropsychologia, 42*(12), 1680-1688.

Wilson, S. M., Rising, K., Stib, M.T., Rapcsak, S.Z., & Beeson, P.M. (2013). Dysfunctional visual word form processing in progressive alexia. *Brain, 136*, 1260-1273.

Wolf, M. (2007). *Proust and the squid: The story and science of the reading brain* (pp. 13-54). New York, NY: HarperCollins Publishers.

Wolfe, J. M. & Bennett, S. (1997). Preattentive object files: Shapeless bundles of basic features. *Vision Research, 37*(1), 25-43.

Zeki, S. (1993). *A vision of the brain.* Cambridge, MA: Blackwell Scientific Publications.

Zihl, J. (2000a). Localised CNS lesions and their effect on visual function. *Optometry Today, 2*(11), 31-32.

TEST BANK

1. The ability to locate objects in space requires the integration of visual input with sensory information from the _____ and _____ systems. (Select 1)
   a. proprioceptive, auditory
   b. sensory, vestibular
   c. vestibular, proprioceptive
   d. auditory, vestibular

2. When we localize a word in relation to other words in a sentence we are using a(n) _____ perspective. (Select 1)
   a. egocentric
   b. allocentric
   c. central
   d. peripheral

3. There are two types of photoreceptor cells in the outermost sensory layer of the retina. Color vision is dependent upon the response of _____ cells to the presence of bright light. _____ cells respond to low light and movement. (Select 1)
   a. rod, cone
   b. light, dark
   c. ciliary, retinal
   d. cone, rod

4. The retina may be divided into three distinct areas. Visual images are the sharpest when they are fixated by the _____ or _____. (Select 1)
   a. fovea, peripheral retina
   b. parafovea, central retina
   c. parafovea, peripheral retina
   d. fovea, central retina

5. Four cranial nerves are involved with vision. They are (Select 1):
   a. II (optic), IV (trochlear), VI (abducens), and VIII (acoustic)
   b. II (optic), III (oculomotor), IV (trochlear), and VI (abducens)
   c. III (oculomotor), VI (abducens), V (trigeminal), and XI (accessory)
   d. I (olfactory), II (optic), III (oculomotor), and IV (trochlear)

6. Visual input from the _____ retina is transmitted through the retinotectal pathway to the _____ in the brainstem. (Select 1)
   a. peripheral, midbrain
   b. peripheral, pulvinar
   c. central, midbrain
   d. central, pulvinar

7. The optic radiation is formed by neural fibers that represent the upper and lower visual fields. Neurons that represent the _____ visual field are in the _____ portion of the optic radiation. Neurons that represent the _____ visual field are in the _____ portion of the optic radiation. (Select 2)
   a. peripheral, central
   b. horizontal, lateral
   c. upper, lower
   d. lower, upper

8. The ventral visual pathway is also called the _____ because it carries information related to the detail of _____. The dorsal visual pathway is also called the _____ because it carries _____ and serves visually guided action. (Select 2)
   a. "where" or "how" visual pathway, spatial information
   b. "where" or "how" visual pathway, object information
   c. "what" visual pathway, objects and faces
   d. "what" visual pathway, facial information

9. The corpus callosum is a bundle of sensory nerve fibers that integrates the functions of the right and left hemispheres. Lesions of the corpus callosum may inhibit the transfer of information from the _____ hemisphere to the _____ hemisphere language areas. (Select 1)
   a. left, right
   b. right, left
   c. left, right
   d. right, right

10. There is a direct correspondence between points on the retina, layers of the lateral geniculate nucleus, points in primary visual cortex and divisions within the visual association cortex. This level of correspondence across structures and cortical locations that process visual information is called _____. (Select 1)
   a. topographic organization
   b. retinotopic organization
   c. tonotopic organization
   d. visual spatial organization

2

Impact of Visual System Dysfunction on Language and Cognition

A Historical Perspective

In this chapter we will examine the ways in which visual sensory and motor dysfunction may negatively impact reading and writing following a neurological event. We will also examine the role working memory plays in reading and spelling. Our understanding of the neuroscience of language and cognition has changed over the past 150 years. Traditional speech therapy assessment is grounded in *localization theory* (Broca, 1861; Naeser & Hayward, 1978), which assumes that there is a direct relationship between cortical structure and function and between locus of lesion and specific language impairment such as the word-finding deficit characteristic of Broca's aphasia. Many formal tests of speech and language function reflect localization theory because they are designed to measure distinct communicative modalities (Goodglass & Kaplan, 1972; Goodglass & Weintraub, 2001; Kertesz, 1982; LaPointe & Horner, 2006).

Multiple Pathways for Audition, Motor Speech, and Vision

Over the past two decades, brain imaging studies have provided strong evidence for separate but interconnected ventral and dorsal neural networks serving audition (Hickok & Poeppel, 2007; Rauschecker, 1998; Rauschecker & Tian, 2000), language, and motor-speech function (Hickok & Poeppel, 2007; Mesulam, 1990; Saur et al., 2008). Neurolinguists Greg Hickok and David Poeppel (2004) have described a dual-stream model of language that includes a cortical conceptual system (semantic) that serves comprehension and a motor speech system where articulatory gestures are shaped to match the phonetic structure of language. For a clear illustration of this model the reader is referred to Hickok and Poeppel (2007). The dorsal auditory stream is located in the posterior part of the Sylvian fissure between the temporal and parietal lobes. It maps sound onto

McMartin Heeringa, H. *The Visual Brain and Peripheral Reading and Writing Disorders: A Guide to Visual System Dysfunction for Speech–Language Pathologists.* (pp. 23-49).

motor movement and serves motor speech acquisition and speech repetition. The ventral auditory stream, including areas of the superior and middle temporal lobe, serves comprehension, mapping sound onto meaning. Likewise, neuropsychological and neuro-optometric studies of vision have identified three primary pathways within the visual system: the ventral, dorsal, and retinotectal pathways (de Gelder, 2010; Milner & Goodale, 2006; Ro & Rafal, 2006; Ungerleider & Mishkin, 1982). The ventral, or central, pathway consciously processes details, identifies objects and flags their purpose and location in relation to other objects within a scene. It is called the *what pathway* because it is involved in form recognition. The dorsal, or peripheral, visual pathway is called the *how pathway* (de Gelder, 2010; Milner & Goodale, 2008) because it subconsciously locates objects and directs movements toward them using egocentric coordinates (i.e., judging the location of objects relative to one's head or torso midline). Finally, the retinotectal pathway transmits visual information from the peripheral retina to the superior colliculi of the midbrain, controlling pupil constriction to manage the amount of light entering the eye. It directs visual attention and controls eye movements to place stimuli at the central retina. Interconnections between these pathways coordinate the different components of vision.

Integrated Cortical Networks

Changes in neuroimaging procedures over the past three decades have allowed for functional neuroimaging of the cortical organization of motor (Calautti & Baron, 2003), cognitive (Munoz-Cespedes, Rios-Lago, & Maestu, 2005), language (Mesulam, 1990; Calvert, Campbell, & Brammer, 2000; Thompson & den Ouden, 2008; Szwed et al, 2012; Woodhead et al., 2013), and visual systems (deGelder, 2010; Golomb & Kanwisher, 2011) and spatial attention networks (Corbetta & Shulman, 2011). The result has been a movement away from localization theory to a theory of brain function that defines networks of functional specialization within multiple, integrated motor and sensory cortical systems (Lewis, Beauchamp, & DeYoe, 2000; McIntosh, 2000; Schuett, Heywood, Kentridge, & Zihl, 2008; Moreno, Schiff, Giacino, Kalmar, & Hirsch, 2010; Corbetta & Shulman, 2011).

Motor and sensory input is integrated within and between different neural systems (e.g. vision and audition) in both a parallel and distributed fashion (Moore, 1986; Goldman-Rakic, 1988; Calvert et al., 2000; de Gelder, 2010). One neural system may have either an enhancing or suppressing effect on the other depending upon the focus of attention and the task being performed. Visual system impairments have the potential to negatively impact both visual language and nonvisual communicative and cognitive functions through the integrated cortical networks that serve these different sensory systems.

Over three decades ago, Josephine Moore (1986), occupational therapist and researcher in the area of visual function in brain injury wrote: "Input from multiple sensory systems is correlated and compared. When there is a lesion, there is a loss of input to the neural centers that feed forward and feed back. This leads to discoordination of temporal and sequential processing of input" (p. 461). Moore advocated for a more holistic view of the brain in rehabilitation that would take into consideration the integrated nature of sensory pathways.

NEUROPLASTICITY

Another important discovery resulting from the evolution of neuroimaging methods is the fact that the injured brain repairs and reorganizes motor (Calautti & Baron, 2003; Kleim et al., 2005; Sakai et al., 1998), visual (Buchel, Coull, & Friston, 1999; Bridge, Thomas, Jhabdi, & Cowey, 2008; Das & Gilbert, 1995; Levi & Polat, 1996; Trauzetti-Klosinski & Reinhard, 1998; Schuett et al., 2008b), motor speech (Petzinger, et al., 2013), auditory (Merzenich et al., 1996; Nichol & Krauss, 2004; Rauschecker, 1999), language (Raichle, et al., 1994; Sims et al., 2002; Sonty et al., 2007;

Temple et al., 2003; Thompson and den Ouden, 2008; Woodhead et al., 2013), attention (Schuett et al., 2008b), memory, and learning functions (Fletcher, Buchel, Josephs, Friston, & Dolan, 1999; Garavan, Kelley, Rosen, Rao, & Stein, 2000).

This cortical reorganization is called *neuroplasticity*. Neuroplastic change occurs in response to learning and in response to therapeutic intervention (Buonomano & Merzenich, 1998; Cramer et al., 2011; Heuninckx, Winderoth, & Swimnen, 2008; Kleim & Jones, 2008).

VISION AND AGING

In the general population, visual changes that significantly impact daily function occur with aging. Studies of the normal aging population show a decline in contrast sensitivity, visual processing speed, sensitivity to light, dynamic vision, near vision, and visual search ability, color vision, visual memory and a reduction in the useful field of view (UFOV), or the amount of visual input that can be grouped and analyzed within one fixation (Bayles et al., 1987; Brussee, van den Berg, van Nispen, & van Rens, 2017; Jackson & Owsley, 2003; Scialfa, Line, & Lyman, 1987). In the context of reading this is referred to as the *perceptual span* (Kim & Lemke, 2016) or *visual span* (Legge et al., 2009). Comparing older readers to younger readers Rayner, Castelhano, and Yang (2009) and Rayner, Slattery, and Belanger, (2010) found that the UFOV for older readers (65 to 81 years) is half that of younger readers (19 to 28 years). Healthy elderly subjects (aged 60 to 84) have shown age-related decline on measures of visual-spatial attention, including cancellation tests (Stone, Halligan, Wilson, Greenwood, & Marshall, 1991). Elderly clients with low vision due to macular degeneration or glaucoma may have impairments in functional vision in activities of daily living such as reading or driving (Jackson & Owsley, 2003; Mahncke, Bronstone, & Merzenich, 2006). Visual sensory impairments in the aging population have also been shown to affect neuropsychological test outcomes (Bertone, Bettinelli, & Faubert, 2007; Powell & Torgerson, 2011; Uzzell, Dolinskas, & Langfit, 1988).

ACQUIRED VISUAL SYSTEM IMPAIRMENT

Visual sensory and motor impairments have frequently been documented in stroke, traumatic brain injury (Farah, 2004; Padula, Shapiro, Jasin, 1988; Gianutsos, 1997), and progressive neurological diseases, including primary progressive aphasia (Sonty et al., 2007) and the dementias (Farah, 2004; Globe, Davis, Schoeberg, & Duvoisin, 1988; Jackson & Owsley, 2003; Milner & Goodale, 2006; Mort & Kennard, 2000; Newcombe & Ratcliff, 1989; Possin, 2010) (see Appendix E). They impede rehabilitation efforts and the recovery of language and cognitive function (Ciuffreda & Kapoor, 2007; Gillen, 2009; Gianutsos, 1997; Kerkhoff & Schenk, 2012; Wolf, 2007), and diminish functional independence (Kerkhoff, 2000; Suter, 2004). Visual system dysfunction can disrupt the bottom-up, peripheral components of visual language processing such as form recognition and adversely affect reading, writing, or spelling and instrumental activities of daily living (Gillen, 2009; Padula & Shapiro, 1988; Schuett et al., 2008b). Therefore, the assessment and treatment of cognitive-communicative dysfunction becomes more challenging in the context of acquired visual impairments. Some clients may appear to have plateaued in their recovery due to undiagnosed visual impairments that are hidden barriers to recovery (Ciuffreda et al., 2007; Gianutsos & Matheson, 1987; Powell & Torgerson, 2011).

LESIONS OF THE VISUAL PATHWAYS

The central visual pathway (i.e., temporoparietal pathway) originates in the cone cells of the central retina where we begin to process visual detail (see Figure 1-5). Lesions of the central pathway result in various deficits of form recognition. These include impaired recognition of faces (i.e., prosopagnosia), places (i.e., topographical agnosia), letters and words (i.e., alexia). The peripheral or dorsal visual stream (i.e., parietooccipital pathway) originates in the rod cells of the peripheral retina. Lesions of the dorsal visual pathway result in right-left confusion; impaired depth perception (i.e., stereoblindness); visuospatial impairment; inability to visually guide reaching and manipulate objects (i.e., optic ataxia); constructional apraxia, which impairs grasping movements (e.g., holding a pencil), tracing, copying, and writing; and the inability to volitionally gaze shift to a target (i.e., ocular apraxia); as well as deficits in figure-ground segregation and motion perception (Caselli, 2000; Kerkhoff, 2000). Finally, the retinotectal pathway controls eye movements that place objects at the central retina where visual acuity is optimal. Visual information from the peripheral retina is transmitted along the retinotectal pathway to the superior colliculi of the midbrain. Following lesions of the superior colliculi individuals are unable to shift visual attention (Zihl, 2000a), leading to deficits in reading and writing. Visual motor and sensory deficits impact reading at a prelexical level (i.e., before phonological or semantic processing occurs) because they interfere with the processing of text.

Eye Movement Disorders

Eye movement is a key component of our ability to see and localize objects. The movements that serve object recognition and visual language function are fixation, saccades, vergence, and accommodation (Gillen, 2009; Sanet & Press, 2011). In accommodation, the eyes converge (i.e., rotate toward midline), the pupils constrict, and the distance of focus is adjusted through contraction of the ciliary muscle. The ciliary muscle is innervated by cranial nerve (CN) III in the midbrain (Gillen, 2009; Hubel, 1995). Convergence is necessary for reading at near distance, writing, and other functional activities that we perform each day such as using a phone, calendar, or computer. When CN III is damaged due to midbrain stroke, traumatic brain injury, or progressive neurological disease, focusing ability is compromised. Subjects complain of slowness in the adjustment of focus as objects approach or when they shift gaze from near to far targets.

Damage to CN III may also cause ptosis, or drooping of the eyelid, and a dilated pupil that leads to complaints of glare (Bhatti, Eisenschenk, Roper, & Guy, 2006; Bhatti, Schmalfuss, Williams, & Quisling, 2003). Reports of blurring, intermittent double vision, headaches, and visual strain are suggestive of accommodative dysfunction (Green et al., 2010a). Both accommodative and vergence difficulties can occur even in mild traumatic brain injury (Green et al., 2010b; Thiagarajan, Ciuffreda, & Ludlam, 2011).

We scan faces, pictures, objects, and print through a series of saccades. This is the process of orienting to the next fixation point and then quickly shifting gaze to that location. A pattern of repetitive saccadic shifts followed by refixation is necessary for reading and other near activities. It is dependent upon a balance between the binocular functions of vergence and accommodation and timely input from brainstem structures that mediate gaze shifting (Suter, 2004). In a review of five recent studies of oculomotor dysfunction, Thiagarajan et al. (2011) found eye movement disorders in 50% to 90% of cases of acquired brain injury; reading difficulty was the most common symptom. When eye movement is impaired, subjects may complain of double vision (Rowe, 2011) or of objects and words blurring (Ciuffreda et al., 2008). Eye movement disorders reduce the frequency and range of saccades for near language activities (Ross & Ma-Wyatt, 2004) and significantly impair the ability to keep objects in focus (Martinez-Conde, 2004; 2006). Visual motor impairments also impede motor planning, leading to the inability to initiate saccades or to delayed saccades (Ciuffreda & Kapoor, 2007; Milner & Goodale, 2006).

Optic Ataxia and Gaze Apraxia

Optic ataxia and gaze apraxia are eye movement disorders associated with lesions of the dorsal visual pathway (Kerkhoff, 2000). People with optic ataxia can identify the location of visual objects but have difficulty with the motor planning and eye-hand coordination involved in reaching for those same objects (Hickok & Poeppel, 2004). Optic ataxia is characterized by impaired reaching across the entire visual field with poor visual guidance of hand and arm movements (Rizzo & Vecera, 2002). Oculomotor apraxia (i.e., gaze apraxia) is the inability to gaze shift toward a new target detected outside the central retinal field (Newcombe & Ratcliff, 1989). This occurs with bilateral occipitoparietal lesions and with damage to connections between primary visual cortex and visual association areas and connections to the frontal eye fields (FEF) (Zihl, 2000b). Gaze apraxia impairs both volitional and reflexive shifts in fixation such as those that occur with reading, writing, copying, or drawing. Formal assessment of language is more challenging because clients have difficulty directing their gaze toward picture and word stimuli and have difficulty maintaining fixation.

Balint Syndrome

Bilateral middle cerebral artery parietal or parieto-occipital lesions produce a unique pattern of deficits known as *Balint syndrome* (Amalnath, Kumar, Deepanjoli, & Dutta, 2014; Kerkhoff, 2000; Newcombe & Ratcliff, 1989; Rizzo and Vecera, 2002; Devinsky & D'Esposito, 2004). These deficits include gaze apraxia, optic ataxia and simultanagnosia, restricted spatial attention (i.e., range of eye movement is diminished), and impaired spatial orientation. The client with Balint syndrome may exhibit wandering gaze, impaired search for visual targets, and have difficulty placing visual targets at the fovea and maintaining gaze fixation. He may need reminders to visually guide his hand movements when writing. A client with bilateral parietooccipital lesions (author observation) described his own attempts to look at what he had written and then begin writing again, as follows: "If I take my eyes off the pencil tip I don't know where I am. It's difficult to read a letter or word and then go back to where I was."

Visual Sensory System Impairment

Visual sensory system impairments include the inability to detect stimuli (e.g., hemianopia, quadrantanopia, perceptual neglect, simultanagnosia, extinction); inability to bring objects into focus (i.e., impaired binocular fusion due to accommodative dysfunction); failure to recognize visual forms such as faces (i.e., prosopagnosia) or color (i.e., central achromatopsia) (Kerkhoff, 2000; Livingstone, 2006); failure to recognize objects (i.e., associative visual agnosia), places (i.e., topographical agnosia), letters or words (i.e., pure alexia) (Farah, 2004); and amblyopia (i.e., loss of both color and form vision) (Fahle & Greenlee, 2003; Hubel, 1995). Related cognitive symptoms include difficulty with sustained visual attention, inability to shift attention between competing visual stimuli, inability to filter out irrelevant visual detail, topographical disorientation, and impaired visual memory. Withdrawal behavior may be noted due to overstimulation. Clients with impairments in both audition and vision (i.e., dual sensory impairment) may be unable to process information simultaneously through more than one sensory modality. They simply cannot look and listen at the same time. Prolonged staring without responding may be noted.

Diminished Visual Acuity

Visual acuity refers to the clarity of vision and the ability to discriminate detail. It is formally tested by occupational therapy or neuro-optometry at near and far distances. Following stroke or traumatic brain injury, performance on visual acuity testing may be reduced due to visual sensory or motor impairments, including deficits in contrast sensitivity (Gillen, 2009) or difficulty localizing and fixating on targets (Zihl, 2000b). Subjective complaints include blurring and difficulty reading. Visual acuity may also be reduced in cases of unilateral or bilateral lesions posterior to

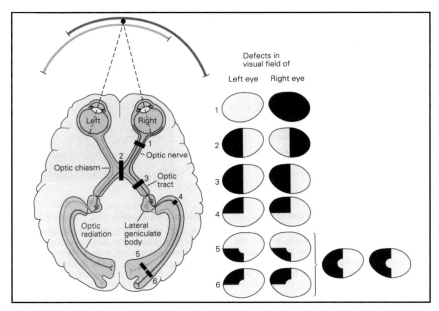

Figure 2-1. Deficits in the visual field produced by lesions at various points in the visual pathway. The level of a lesion can be determined by the specific deficit in the visual field. In the diagram of the cortex, the numbers along the visual pathway indicate the sites of lesions. The deficits that result from lesions at each site are shown in the visual field maps on the right as black areas. Deficits in the visual field of the left eye represent what an individual would *not see* with the right eye closed rather than deficits of the left visual hemifield. (Reprinted with permission from Kandel, E. R., Schwartz, J. H., & Jessel, T. M. [2000], *Principles of neural science* [4th ed]. New York, NY: McGraw-Hill Education.)

the optic chiasm (Kerkhoff, 2000) (Figure 2-1). Loss of vision in the central visual field results in a total loss of visual acuity (Margolis, 2011) because central vision is necessary for form recognition and seeing objects in detail.

Impaired Depth Perception

Because our eyes are offset in the horizontal plane, each eye has a slightly different field of view. The difference in these two images is called *binocular disparity* (Gonzalez, Relova, Prieto, & Peleteiro, 2005; Ratcliff & Ross, 1981; Wheatstone, 1838). Monocular cues such as texture, relative size, and linear perspective, are combined with information on binocular disparity to achieve the perception of depth. This is called *binocular fusion*. This information is integrated through the corpus callosum allowing the viewer to judge distance from an egocentric perspective (relative to midline of the retina, head or torso) (Barbato & Addington, 2014; Brouwer, van Ee, & Schwarzbach, 2005; Miller et al., 1999; Mittenberg, Choi, & Apple, 2000). Well-coordinated eye-teaming movements (i.e., vergence) and the ability to focus at near and far distances (i.e., accommodation) are foundation skills for depth perception (Powell & Torgerson, 2011). A binocular fusion deficit impairs reading and writing and can result in letter or word omissions, duplications, and confusion about the sequence of printed letters and words. Lesions of the visual association cortex (i.e., Brodmann, 19) and temporal and parietal lobes cause deficits in depth perception (Kerkhoff, 2000).

Low Blink Rate

Eye blinks occur reflexively 10 to 15 times/minute to maintain corneal moistness and oxygenation. During blinking, vision is suppressed for 100 to 150 milliseconds (Burr, 2005). Bristow, Frith, and Rees (2005) used functional magnetic resonance imaging to measure the cortical response to visual input in the context of voluntary blinking. They found that voluntary blinking increased the cortical response in the medial parietooccipital region. Tse, Baumgartner, and Greenlee (2010) studied the response of the visual cortex to microsaccades (see page 8), voluntary saccades, and eye blinks, each of which changed the input to retinal ganglion cells in a transient manner. The authors found a related transient increase in the response of the visual cortex as input to the retinal ganglion cells was refreshed through blinking. Tasks with higher cognitive load, including mathematical problem solving or memorization, are associated with increased rate of blinking (Holland & Tarlow, 1972). Low blink rate or staring behavior is a symptom of post-trauma vision syndrome, a constellation of visual symptoms that occur following brain injury (Padula et al., 1988). Low blink rate also contributes to dry eye syndrome (Abelson, 2011).

Impaired Contrast Sensitivity

The neural response to contrast between light and dark reveals the borders and edges of forms. This allows the viewer to distinguish one object from another (Farah, 2000; Kandel, Schwartz, & Jessel, 1995). A reduction in contrast sensitivity occurs with normal aging (Brussee et al., 2017). In stroke and traumatic brain injury, post-chiasmic lesions (see Figure 2-1) impair spatial and temporal contrast sensitivity, and the perception of depth and distance (Kerkhoff, 2000). Deficits in contrast sensitivity are associated with reading difficulty and lower functional independence scores; however, they may not be detected without a thorough visual function examination (dos Santos & Andrade, 2012).

Visual Field Loss and Reading

Visual field loss is a deficit in light perception or loss of vision in a portion of the visual field. Following stroke, tumor, or traumatic brain injury, partial loss of the visual fields may occur on the same (i.e., ipsilateral) or the opposite side (i.e., contralateral) to the lesion. Rayner (1998) divided the retina into three distinct areas (see Chapter 1 Figure 1-1; fovea = numbers 1 to 4, parafovea = numbers 5 to 8, and peripheral retina = numbers 9 to 12). The right parafoveal field processes details such as word length and word boundaries, guides eye movement, and is important in the recognition of whole words, the spaces between words, and word length (Gillen 2009; Leff et al., 2004; Zihl, 2000b). The ability to view the word to the right of the fixated word (i.e., the word that falls in the right parafoveal region) is crucial to the reading process (Rayner, 2009; Schuett et al., 2008b).

Citing several studies of reading, Zihl (2000c) has stated that "… earlier and recent observations strongly suggest that parafoveal field loss affects reading at the sensory level; it prevents the patient perceiving a word as a whole and impairs the visual guidance of eye movements." Therefore, the processing of graphic input by the parafoveal visual field is very important in reading.

The ability to process the beginning of words is tied to the ability to access the orthographic lexicon (i.e., mental lexicon) and the ability to choose among a group of words that share the same initial letters (White, Johnson, Liversedge, & Rayner, 2008). Fixation location and duration are also impacted by the ability to process the beginning of words (Hand et al, 2012). Readers with hemianopia of the left visual field have difficulty shifting gaze back to the left margin and tend to omit word prefixes (Schuett et al., 2008b; Zihl, 2000b). To read English text at a normal rate, readers also need to be able to detect up to 15 letters to the right of the fixation point (Rayner et al., 2010). In cases of right hemianopia with a loss of central vision the reader is unable to preprogram eye movements to the right (McConkie & Rayner, 1976; Suter & Margolis, 2005). Right parafoveal field loss results in a significantly higher ratio of saccades (i.e., gaze shifts) to words compared to normal readers. Rather than fixating to the left of the middle of words, which is the normal pattern, the reader with right hemianopia tends to fixate at the beginning of words, and smaller words are more likely to be fixated (Rayner, 1979). Symptoms include slower reading, misinterpretation of text, diminished ability to anticipate words and ideas, impaired reading comprehension, and impaired memory for written material. Clients with unilateral and bilateral field loss will typically produce eye movements that are inadequate to compensate for their visual field loss (i.e., hypometric saccades) in the ipsilateral, contralateral, or both directions, and may report slow visual processing (Zihl, 2000b). The reader is referred to Pula and Yuen (2017) for a detailed description of the various types of visual field loss and their associated lesions.

Blindsight/Cortical Blindness

Despite the inability to consciously identify colors, objects, or words, some subjects with central visual field deficits due to lesions in the primary visual cortex retain the subconscious visual ability to respond to motion in their blind fields, localize visual targets using saccades or by pointing, and detect the directional orientation of an object (Leh, Johansen-Berg, & Pitto, 2006). This residual visual ability in the absence of conscious vision is called *blindsight* (Campion, Latto, & Smith, 1983; Giaschi et al., 2003; Pöppel, Held, & Frost, 1973; Weiskrantz, Warrington, Sanders, & Marshall, 1974; Zeki & Ffytche, 1998). Blindsight has been reported in cases of hemispherectomy (Perenin & Jeannerod, 1978; Ptito et al., 1991), stroke (Fendrich, Wessinger, & Gazzinga, 1992; Sahraie et al., 2003), anoxia (Milner et al., 1991), and traumatic brain injury (Pöppel et al., 1973). Bilateral ischemic lesions of the occipital lobe are associated with cortical blindness (Glisson, 2014), which has been attributed to subconscious residual visual ability in the dorsal visual pathway in cases where central vision is lost or severely impaired (Dehaene, 2014; James, Culham, Humphrey, Milner, & Goodale, 2003). Neuroimaging studies of hemianopic clients also suggest that the superior colliculus of the midbrain may play a role in residual vision in cases of blindsight (de Gelder, 2010). It has been proposed that in such cases the superior colliculus provides the primary sensory input to the dorsal visual pathway for stimulus detection (Ajina & Rees, 2011; Milner & Goodale, 2006).

Impaired Spatial Perception, Attention, and Neglect

Impaired Spatial Perception

All visual information is segregated by the eye of origin and is organized retinotopically. This means that there is a direct correspondence between points on the retina, layers of the lateral geniculate nucleus, points in the primary visual cortex, and divisions within the visual association cortex (Baker, 2000; Tong, 2003). When we move our eyes the cortical spatial map that localizes objects in relation to one another and in relation to body position is continually updated. Interconnections between areas of the visual cortex that represent midline ensure that our view is uninterrupted as our gaze shifts from left to right across midline. Spatial mapping has been found to occur at the level of the parietal cortex, visual association cortex, superior colliculi of the midbrain and frontal eye fields (Merriam & Colby, 2005). Spatial perception is also important in reading because we use it to determine which direction letters and numbers should face (Papagno, 2002) and for judging size differences (Farah, Hammond, Levine, & Calvanio, 1988). Lesions that impact the coordination of eye movements, produce visual field defects, or interfere with binocular fusion (i.e., cortical binding of the two offset images) lead to impairments in spatial perception and depth perception (Sanet and Press, 2011; Schaadt, Brandt, Kraft, & Kerkhoff, 2015).

Hemispatial Neglect

In hemispatial neglect there is typically a failure to search for and recognize stimuli in the visual field contralateral to the lesion. One recent study reported the prevalence of neglect symptoms following stroke to be 3 to 5 million cases each year (Corbetta, Kincade, Lewis, Snuder, & Sapir, 2005). Chronic neglect occurs in approximately one-third of cases (Kerkhoff & Schenk, 2012). Patterns of hemispatial neglect differ within and between subjects and have been documented in lesions in diverse areas of the cortex (Parton, Malhorta, & Husain, 2004; Verdon et al., 2010). Reports of the prevalence of unilateral spatial neglect (USN) are inconsistent across studies because of differences in time post-onset; lack of consistency in testing instruments and study design (Bowen et al., 1999); and the fact that neglect is a heterogenous disorder that is observed in tasks across multiple domains (e.g., motor, sensory, language) (Azouvi et al., 2006; Saj, Verdon, Vocat, & Vuilleumier, 2011).

Halligan, Fink, Marshall, and Wallar (2003) systematically tested subjects with visual neglect over two decades. The authors concluded that the variability in presentation of visual neglect may be accounted for by impairments in different *spatial reference frames* (see also Kleinman et al., 2007; Nichelli, Venneri, Pentore, & Cubelli, 1993). Judgements about location and spatial orientation depend upon whether the viewer's frame of reference is *egocentric* or *allocentric* (Halligan et al., 2003; Milner & Goodale, 2006; Marsh & Hillis, 2008; Reinhart, Schindler, & Kerkhoff, 2011). When the frame of spatial reference is egocentric, object midline is perceived relative to the center of the viewer's retina, head, or body, and stimuli in the contralateral field are neglected. This conclusion is supported by studies of neglect in copying and drawing (Halligan et al., 2003; Hillis et al., 2005), reading (Caramazza & Hillis, 1990; Humphreys & Riddoch, 1995), and neuropsychological test batteries (Medina et al., 2009; Verdon et al., 2010).

With an allocentric frame of reference the location of one object is determined relative to the location of other objects in a scene and neglect occurs within objects across the visual field. The studies cited previously referenced two types of allocentric reference frames:

- *Object-centered*, where the left side of a word is determined relative to its initial letter
- *Stimulus-centered*, where words are viewed as objects and midline is determined by the center of the object regardless of its orientation (e.g., vertical, horizontal, mirror image) or placement within the visual field (Table 2-1). Medina et al. (2009) found that some individuals with object-centered right neglect miss letters and syllables at the ending of words when reading, spelling aloud, and listening to words spelled aloud. Oral sentence reading distinguishes *viewer-centered neglect* from object- and stimulus-centered neglect (Hillis, 2006).

Attention and Hemispatial Neglect

Corbetta and Shulman (2011) studied attention and the physiological signs of left neglect. They described two interactive but distinct networks that modulate attention and awareness:

- A dorsal frontoparietal attention network involved with spatial functions
- A ventral frontoparietal attention network involved with nonspatial functions.

Their findings are outlined in Table 2-2. The authors hypothesized that left hemispatial neglect results from the reduced interactions of these two attention networks following a right hemisphere neurological event. While neglect of the left visual field is a familiar outcome of a right cerebrovascular accident (CVA), historically it has been assumed that neglect of the right visual field following left hemisphere CVA is rare (Behrmann, Black, McKeefm & Barton, 2002; Beis et al., 2004; Corbetta and Shulman, 2011; Gillen, 2009). In some cases, errors occurring in the right half of words have been attributed to aphasic disturbance (e.g., naming errors) rather than to visuospatial impairment or neglect. The similarity to errors in left neglect dyslexia is overlooked (Berndt et al., 2005).

Most studies of unilateral spatial neglect (USN) focus on cases of right hemisphere stroke (Behrmann et al., 2002; Parton et al., 2004; Vallar, 2007; Verdon, Schwartz, Lorblad, Hauert, & Vuilleumier, 2010) and do not include in-depth measures of text reading (Beschin, Cisari, Cubelli, & Della Sala, 2014) or of writing. However, in a magnetic resonance imaging study, Kleinman et al. (2007) examined USN in 47 right-handed cases of acute left hemisphere stroke. By including word copying tasks in their attention battery, they found a higher frequency of right hemispatial neglect than is typically reported. The authors concluded that in cases of USN, allocentric (i.e., object-based) errors occur more frequently in left hemisphere stroke, whereas egocentric (i.e., viewer-based) errors occur more often in right hemisphere stroke (see Table 2-1). They proposed that spatial attention is directed by the left hemisphere across single objects such as words, and is directed globally and bilaterally relative to a viewer-centered midline by the right hemisphere. These findings were consistent with those of an earlier study by Edmans and Lincoln (1987) in

TABLE 2-1

THREE TYPES OF LEFT VISUAL SPATIAL NEGLECT AND ASSOCIATED ERROR PATTERNS BASED ON SPATIAL REFERENCE FRAMES

EGOCENTRIC REFERENCE FRAME		ALLOCENTRIC REFERENCE FRAME			
Viewer-Centered Neglect		*Object-Centered Neglect*		*Stimulus-Centered Neglect*	
Midline is defined by center of viewer's retina, head, or body. Entire stimulus is neglected if it is presented to the left visual field.		For objects with a canonical orientation (e.g. words, maps, or flags), midline is defined by the center of the target regardless of its orientation or location in relation to the viewer. Errors occur at the beginning of words in all positions (mirror-image words; words rotated 90 degrees, etc.) (see below)		The left side of word and object stimuli is neglected, whether the stimulus is presented to the left or right side of the body, or at midline. Unlike object-centered neglect, in stimulus-centered neglect the left side of mirror-image words or objects is neglected.	
LEFT FIELD	RIGHT FIELD	LEFT FIELD	RIGHT FIELD	LEFT FIELD	RIGHT FIELD
...that there are two interactive but distinct networks that modulate attention and awareness: a dorsal frontoparietal attention network is involved with spatial functions and a ventral frontoparietal attention network involved with nonspatial functions.		LIGHTHOUSE (spanning)			LIGHTHOUSE (right-aligned)
		LIGHTHOUSE (mirror-reversed, spanning)		LIGHTHOUSE	
					LIGHTHOUSE (mirror-reversed, right-aligned)
		LIGHTHOUSE (vertical)	LIGHTHOUSE (vertical)	LIGHTHOUSE (mirror-reversed)	
				LIGHTHOUSE (right-aligned)	
				LIGHTHOUSE (mirror-reversed)	

Adapted from Medina, J., Kannan, V., Pawlak, M. A., Kleinman, J. T., Newhart, M., Davis, C., ... Hillis, A. E. (2009). Neural substrates of visuospatial processing in distinct reference frames: Evidence from unilateral spatial neglect. *Journal of Cognitive Neuroscience*, *21*(11), 2073-2084.

which word copying was more sensitive to right hemispatial neglect in left hemisphere stroke. In light of these findings, assessment for USN should be carried out in equal measure with both left hemisphere and right hemisphere clients; testing should be expanded to include more challenging measures of reading and writing or copying; and therapeutic interventions for vision-related language impairment should target the specific type of inattention or neglect reflected in the individual's pattern of errors.

Corbetta and Shulman (2011) have stated, "Damage to right hemisphere ventral regions...... hypo-activates the right hemisphere, reducing interactions between the ventral and dorsal attention network and between regions of the ipsilesional (right) dorsal network. The result is unbalanced inter-hemispheric physiological activity in the dorsal network...... in a direction that favors the left hemisphere." In other words, lesions in the right TPJ, IPL/STG, VFC, or IFG/MFG result in

TABLE 2-2		
DORSAL AND VENTRAL FRONTOPARIETAL ATTENTION NETWORKS ARE DISRUPTED IN LEFT NEGLECT		
	DORSAL FRONTOPARIETAL ATTENTION NETWORK	**VENTRAL FRONTOPARIETAL ATTENTION NETWORK**
CORTICAL LOCATIONS OF VISUAL ATTENTION NETWORKS	• Medial intraparietal sulcus (MIPS) • Superior longitudinal fasciculus (SLF), precuneus • Supplementary eye fields (SEF) • Frontal eye fields (FEF)	• Temporoparietal junction (TPJ) • Inferior parietal lobule/superior temporal gyrus (IPL/STG) • Visual frontal cortex (VFC) • Inferior frontal gyrus/medial frontal gyrus (IFG/MFG)
CORTICAL ORGANIZATION	• Symmetrically organized in the right and left hemisphere	• Lateralized primarily to the right hemisphere
LESION SITES		• (TPJ), (IPL/STG), (VFC) and (IFG/MFG)
TYPICAL DEFICITS IN RIGHT HEMISPHERE DYSFUNCTION	• Spatial attention bias toward the ipsilesional field • Reduced responsiveness • Saliency deficit: Failure to ignore irrelevant stimuli—*can't see the forest for the trees*; fails to attend to stimuli that are relevant to the task they are currently engaged in	• Reduced interhemispheric interaction between ventral and dorsal attention networks and between components of the right (ipsilesional) dorsal frontoparietal attention network • Diminished arousal and vigilance • Deficit in reorienting: Inability to disengage attention from stimuli in the ipsilesional field and to redirect attention to stimuli in the contralateral field • Deficit in detecting novel events that are behaviorally relevant (e.g., tendency to refixate words/objects rather than to respond to novel stimuli)
Adapted from Corbetta, M. & Shulman, G. (2011). Spatial neglect and attention networks. *Annual Review of Neuroscience, 34,* 569-599.		

reduced activation of the right hemisphere leading to disruption of both ventral and dorsal fronto-parietal attention networks (see Table 2-2) resulting in impaired attention to the left hemispatial field.

Agnosia

Visual agnosia is the failure to recognize objects despite normal acuity (Fahle & Greenlee, 2003; Gillen, 2009). It is historically defined according to two subtypes: *apperceptive agnosia* and *associative agnosia* (Farah, 2000; Lissauer, 1890). In apperceptive agnosia, individuals can identify and describe features such as lines, colors, and textures, but are unable to bind them into recognizable objects. They are unable to recognize numbers, letters, or words. In associative agnosia, basic perception is intact. The individual is able to see, match, and copy basic forms but does not associate them with meaning. In simultanagnosia, the individual cannot identify or point to a single object within a group of objects (Amalnath et al., 2014; Farah, 2004; Gillen, 2009). He or she does not recognize whole scenes because he or she only sees one object at a time.

Dorsal and Ventral Simultanagnosia

Farah (2004) describes two types of simultanagnosia: ventral and dorsal simultanagnosia. Lesions within the posterior temporal or temporo-occipital cortex result in ventral simultanagnosia. There is awareness of the presence of more than one object, but an inability to recognize or focus on more than one object at a time. What the viewer perceives is determined by the number of objects, rather than their size or position. Reading is impaired in cases of ventral simultanagnosia due to the inability to attend to more than one letter at a time (Bauer, 2012).

Dorsal simultanagnosia occurs with bilateral lesions that typically include the parietal and superior occipital regions (Amalnath et al., 2014; Farah, 2004). Clients with dorsal simultanagnosia are unable to rapidly shift their visual attention between objects. They may gaze at a single object for a prolonged period of time. Once their gaze is fixed, dorsal simultanagnosics are unaware of other objects or parts of objects. For example, the client with dorsal simultanagnosia is unable to identify and locate both knife and spoon placed side-by-side when eating. Objects appear to fade out and reappear. This phenomenon is reported by clients with visual system dysfunction during administration of the Assessment of Language-Related Functional Activities counting money subtest (Baines, Martin, McMartin Heeringa, 1999) (author observation) (see page 57). Farah (2004) states: "It seems likely that visual disorientation is secondary to, and an inevitable consequence of, the attentional disorder in dorsal simultanagnosia … The inability of dorsal simultanagnosics to attend to two separate locations will therefore be expected to impair localization" (p. 32).

Prosopagnosia

Prosopagnosia impairs the ability to bind facial features into recognizable faces, although the ability to recognize objects may be preserved (Farah, 2004). Some individuals see facial features as if they are drawn in with chalk or blurred. They may rely on hair color or voice recognition to identify family members and close acquaintances. Prosopagnosia occurs with bilateral lesions of the lingual and fusiform gyri (fusiform face area) in the right visual association cortex (Burton, Press, Keenan, & O'Connor, 2002; Devinsky & D'Esposito, 2004; Kanwisher, McDermott, & Chun, 1997) and with progressive lesions of the right temporal lobe (Evans, Heggs, Antoun, & Hodges, 1995).

Acquired Dyslexias

Visual system impairments diminish bottom-up visual processes such as visual acuity, contrast sensitivity, spatial perception, and attention, that are active at the earliest stages of reading (Leff et al., 2000). The reading disorders that result are called *peripheral dyslexias* (Vallar, Burani, & Arduino, 2010) to differentiate them from central reading disorders such as aphasia and phonological or surface alexia (see Table 2-3). An individual client may present with more than one type of peripheral dyslexia such as hemianopic dyslexia and pure alexia. When lesions are extensive and involve the left fusiform gyrus (i.e., visual word form area) and the occipital lobes, signs of both central and peripheral language impairment may be noted (Leff & Schofield, 2010).

Letter-by-Letter Reading Strategy

Lesions of the central (i.e., ventral) visual pathway produce impairments in the recognition of letters and words (i.e., alexia), static forms (i.e., agnosia), and faces (i.e., prosopagnosia) despite normal visual acuity (Fahle and Greenlee, 2003; Gillen, 2009). Agnosia for letters and words limits reader access to the *orthographic lexicon*, the long-term memory for words accessed through phonological and visual orthographic input (Beeson, Rewega, Vail, & Rapcsak, 2000). A commonly used compensatory strategy is *letter-by-letter reading* (LBL). This is the slow, effortful decoding of each letter in a word. Letters and their associated phonemes are identified sequentially and held in working memory (see following) until the word can be identified (Farah, 2004; Lott, Carney, Glezer, & Friedman, 2010; Kim, Rapcsak, Anderson, & Beeson, 2011; Kim, Rising, Rapcsak, & Beeson, 2015; Schuett et al., 2008). LBL reading is associated with pure alexia (i.e., alexia without agraphia), multimodal alexia, and aphasia and the central language disorders of surface alexia and surface agraphia (Table 2-4). When LBL readers read text their eye movement patterns are significantly altered, with more frequent fixations and regressive saccades, and longer fixations in comparison with normal readers, while eye movements in visual search tasks are normal (Behrmann, Shomstein, Black, & Barton, 2001). One particularly insightful client with bilateral parietooccipital strokes (author observation) described his own version of LBL reading:

"I'm having an awful time reading. I'm spending too much time figuring out what a letter is. I read the letters first and then put them together into a word. I read letter-by-letter instead of trying to do it in one gulp."

Dehaene (2009) reports that pure alexics show a delay of 5 to 10 seconds to recognize a single word using LBL reading. This is in sharp contrast to the 150 milliseconds in takes for word recognition in the normal population (Wolf, 2007).

Inner Speech, Working Memory, and Spelling

Reading and oral and written spelling require the quick, conscious processing of orthographic and phonological elements of language and the short-term storage of sequences of letters, sounds, and words. The *graphemic buffer* is a component of working memory. Theoretically, it provides a kind of workspace for written spelling. As words are retrieved from the orthographic lexicon, letters are identified sequentially and stored in the graphemic buffer, also called the *visuospatial sketchpad*. A graphemic buffer deficit results in more frequent writing and spelling errors on longer words (i.e., the *word length effect*; Caramazza, Miceli, Villa, & Romani, 1987; Cloutman et al., 2009) because letters that have been identified slip from memory and the spelling process must begin again and again (Tainturier & Rapp, 2004).

The phonological component of working memory involves the temporary storage of auditory traces within the *phonological buffer* (Baddeley, 2012). Inner speech (i.e., subvocal articulation or articulatory rehearsal) is the ability to think in words. Inner speech utilizes auditory traces that are held in the phonological buffer and rehearsed while the individual completes a single task such as decoding letters to decipher a word, remembering a phone number or email address long enough to write it down, working through a mental math problem, or alternating between two different tasks (Baddeley, 2007; Emerson & Miyake, 2003; Laurent et al., 2016). A deficit in articulatory rehearsal means the individual cannot recall more than one or two phonemes at a time and is thus unable to blend sounds into words. Geva, Bennett, Warburton, and Patterson (2011) demonstrated that inner speech is impaired in some persons with aphasia, but is not positively correlated with overt speech or verbal fluency.

	TABLE 2-3
	PERIPHERAL READING DISORDERS AND TYPICAL ERROR PATTERNS
HEMIANOPIC DYSLEXIA	• Disordered saccades • Excessive fixations and regressions with slower reading rate • Readers omit parts of words or substitute words either to the left or right of midline, depending upon the side of the field cut. • Particular to persons who have a macular-splitting hemianopia (Woodhead et al., 2015). • The reader exhibits a visual sensory deficit with failure to adapt his or her visual scan pattern to visual field loss (Schuett et al., 2008).
NEGLECT DYSLEXIA	• Words, syllables, or entire lines of print may be omitted. • Words may be substituted or added. • Depending upon viewer's spatial frame of reference (egocentric/allocentric; object-centered/ stimulus-centered), errors may occur to the left or right of midline, or across the visual field. • Error patterns reflect changes in spatial reference frames. • In left neglect dyslexia, errors occur at the left margin and at midline; prefixes and initial letters are omitted or substituted (Reinhart et al., 2011). • Neglect dyslexia is found in subjects who have hemispatial neglect of the contralateral field in combination with an altered oculomotor pattern across the entire field (see Table 2-1) (Medina et al., 2009).
ATTENTIONAL DYSLEXIA	• Longer fixations, excessive fixations are noted. • The same passage is read multiple times. • Able to read single letters but not a series of letters • Able to read single words, but not words in a series • Letters from neighboring words may be combined although some attribute this to "crowding" rather than attention (Pelli et al, 2004). • The reader is unable to encode letter positions because he or she cannot attend to more than one object (letter or word) at a time. • Alternatively, Davis and Coltheart (2002) suggest that a reader with attentional dyslexia cannot narrow his or her window of attention to limit interference from words that flank target words.
	(continued)

Table 2-3 (continued)
Peripheral Reading Disorders and Typical Error Patterns

ALEXIA WITHOUT AGRAPHIA (PURE ALEXIA)	• Readers are unable to identify letters and/or words. They use the LBL reading strategy. • Longer words are harder to identify (Kim et al., 2011). • A high percentage of cases of pure alexia have a right homonymous visual field deficit (Leff et al., 2001). • Error pattern is attributed to a right field deficit and damage to the visual word form area (Pflugshaupt et al., 2009). • Alexia without agraphia is associated with lesions of the left occipital temporal sulcus in the area of the fusiform gyrus (McCandliss et al., 2003). • Temporo-occipital lesions; the disruption of input from occipital cortex through inferior longitudinal fasciculus to the Visual Word Form Area (at the left lateral occipitotemporal sulcus) • Lexical decision making and semantic categorization may demonstrate partial access to semantic info. • Word frequency and imageability affect word recognition (Kim et al., 2011).
GLOBAL ALEXIA (MULTIMODAL ALEXIA)	• Letter recognition is poor. • Many letter naming errors, thus unable to use LBL reading strategy. (Lott et al., 2010) • May be able to write but cannot read own writing (Lott et al., 2010). • Error pattern is attributed to visual-verbal disconnection (i.e., unable to retrieve letter names from letter forms). • In a more severe form with kinesthetic-verbal disconnection, client is unable to retrieve letter names by tracing them (Kim et al., 2011). • Associated with lesions of the left hemisphere perisylvian region
KINESTHETIC ALEXIA	• Impaired access to graphic motor programs that direct letter writing (Kim et al., 2011) • Lesion to left (SPL)/intraparietal sulcus.

Acquired Peripheral Agraphia/Dysgraphia

Acquired peripheral dysgraphias are attributed to loss of access to specific motor sequences associated with letter formation (i.e., the size and order of the strokes), as in apraxic agraphia (de Rodrigues, de Fontoura, & Salles, 2014; Planton, Jucla, Roux, Demonet, 2013), discoordinated eye-hand movements, as in spatial agraphia or constructional apraxia (Purcell, Turkeltaub, Eden, & Rapp, 2011; Ullrich & Roeltgen, 2012), visual motor impairments (e.g., disruption of saccades, dysconjugate gaze), visuospatial impairment (i.e., coordinating egocentric and allocentric frames of

	TABLE 2-4
	CENTRAL AND PERIPHERAL WRITING DISORDERS
	ERROR PATTERNS IN PERIPHERAL WRITING DISORDERS
APRAXIC AGRAPHIA	Poorly formed letters in spontaneous writing or in copying due to a deficit in motor programming. Oral spelling is intact. It is associated with lesions of Brodmann's area 7 and 40 (de Rodrigues et al., 2014; Planton et al., 2013).
SPATIAL AGRAPHIA	Also called visuospatial agraphia, constructional agraphia, or afferent dysgraphia. Letter components or strokes are malformed, with duplication of letter strokes, writing uphill or downhill, or extra spaces between letters. It is associated with lesions of the nondominant parietal or frontal lobe, or alternatively with cerebellar lesions (Ullrich & Roeltgen, 2012).
ALLOGRAPHIC AGRAPHIA	Inability to write or copy letters; or may be able to write in upper but not lowercase letters; may be able to print but not write in cursive. An impairment in the graphemic buffer results in an allographic processing deficit (impaired working memory for spelling, writing, and typing). Words retrieved from long-term memory cannot be held in the graphemic buffer long enough to convert them to letter names (in oral spelling), or to graphemes (in writing) (de Rodrigues et al., 2014; Purcell et al., 2011a). Allographic agraphia occurs in left parieto-occipital infarcts (Davies et al, 1997; Black et al, 1989).
ALLOGRAPHIC BUFFER DEFICIT	Mixed use of upper- and lowercase letters, or mixed use of cursive and print, within the same word. Associated with lesions of the left temporo-parietal-occipital cortex (Menichelli et al, 2008).
MULTIMODAL DYSGRAPHIA	Visual-verbal and kinesthetic-verbal disconnections impairs letter recognition for reading and writing. The kinesthetic letter tracing strategy (e.g., on paper, in the air, in their hand) used in LBL reading is not immediately useful but may improve with training. Attributed to damage to the temporal occipital lobes, parietal lobe, and white matter pathways of the occipital lobe that interfere with the transfer of visual input to the right hemisphere across the corpus callosum to the left-hemisphere language areas (Kim et al., 2011).
NEGLECT DYSGRAPHIA	Errors in writing and spelling occur on the contralesional side of words (Kleinman et al., 2007).

(continued)

reference), and visual sensory deficits (e.g., visual field loss, impaired contrast sensitivity, impaired form or color vision).

Allographic Dysgraphia

Some clients also have difficulty converting abstract letter identities to specific allographs (i.e., assigning a letter name, case, and font to form a letter; allographic agraphia) (Davies, Coughlin, & Ellis, 1997; de Rodrigues et al., 2014; Menichelli, Rapp, & Semenza, 2008). This results in a

TABLE 2-4 (CONTINUED)	
CENTRAL AND PERIPHERAL WRITING DISORDERS	
	ERROR PATTERNS IN CENTRAL WRITING DISORDERS
SEMANTIC AGRAPHIA	Written responses consist of semantic jargon, with inability to write with meaning; some subjects will write pseudowords or nonwords and irregularly spelled words correctly. Lesions are in the lexical route where semantic knowledge is disconnected from the lexical system; associated with aphasia, alexia, and ideomotor apraxia (Ullrich & Roeltgen, 2012).
LEXICAL AGRAPHIA (SURFACE AGRAPHIA)	More errors in writing familiar words with irregular spellings or heterographs (i.e., sound the same but with different spellings) than when writing nonwords or pseudowords (Magrassi et al., 2010). Irregular words are spelled phonologically (e.g., "kome" for "comb"). Lesions are in the lexical-orthographic (lexical) route; occurs often with aphasia (Ullrich & Roeltgen, 2012) and with extrasylvian lesions of left hemisphere involving the angular gyrus, posterior lateral, and ventral temporal cortex (Rapcsak & Beeson, 2002).
DEEP AGRAPHIA	Errors are semantically-related whole words (e.g., writing "flight" when the stimulus was "propeller" (Ullrich & Roeltgen, 2012). Lesions impact both the nonlexical phonological route and the semantic route.
PHONOLOGICAL AGRAPHIA	More errors in writing unfamiliar words and nonwords or pseudowords; errors resemble the target word and reflect impairment in the phonological route; similar to phonological alexia in the inability to convert phonemes to graphemes in nonwords (Magrassi et al., 2010); occurs often with aphasia (Ullrich & Roeltgen, 2012).
MIXED OR GLOBAL DYSGRAPHIA	Limited ability to write regular words with marked difficulty writing pseudowords (de Rodrigues et al., 2014). Lesions impact phonological and lexical routes.

significant impairment in spelling, writing, or typing longer words (i.e., word length effect). Individuals with peripheral dysgraphia may see "illusory conjunctions" (Treisman & Schmidt, 1982) when they are copying letters that contain more than one feature (line, curve, conjunction of two lines). Illusory conjunctions occur when a letter appears to be formed by the features of several different letters. Pelli et al., (2004) attribute illusory conjunctions to "crowding", which Pelli et al., (2007) define as "excessive feature integration, inappropriately including extra features that spoil recognition of the target object." In milder cases of dysgraphia, the client may selectively be able to write some words in capital letters or in lowercase, in print or cursive (Menichelli et al., 2008; Purcell, Turkeltaub, et al., 2011). When letter selection or formation is delayed, letter identities and sequences of letters may not be retained long enough to write them (Baddeley, 2003; Lambert et al., 2007; Menichelli, Machetta, Zadini, & Semenza, 2012; Purcell, Napoliello, & Eden, 2011) (see Table 2-4).

Central Dysgraphia

Central dysgraphias, on the other hand, are written spelling disorders attributed to impaired access to the orthographic lexicon (i.e., long-term memory for learned words) through semantic, phonological, or lexical-orthographic routes (Rapp, 2002). The correct spelling of words is determined at the level of the phonological or graphemic buffer (i.e., working memory for spelling), and then linked up with motor speech and written motor planning systems (Ullrich & Roeltgen, 2012).

Alexia with Agraphia

Lesions of the temporal, occipital, and parietal lobe and white matter pathways of the occipital lobe interfere with the transfer of visual input from the nondominant hemisphere across the corpus callosum to the left hemisphere–dominant language areas (Kim et al., 2011) resulting in alexia with agraphia, also called *multimodal dysgraphia*. The subject is neither able to recognize letter and word forms, nor write letters or words. When letter naming is also impaired, the client is unable to use the LBL strategy to decode words. When a lesion impacts the motor planning aspect of writing, the client may substitute letters that are produced with a similar pattern of written strokes such as T and L, or E and F (Menichelli et al., 2008; Rapp, 2002).

In summary, current theory of brain function presumes that focal lesions affect cortical connections across networks of functional specialization (Carter, Shulman, & Corbetta, 2012; Moore, 1986). Visual system impairments diminish bottom-up, visual processes such as visual acuity, contrast sensitivity, spatial perception, and attention, at the earliest stages of reading (Leff et al., 2000). They have the potential to impact other language, cognitive, and visual networks that feed forward and backward as new information is acquired and combined with previously learned details. Subjects may have difficulty localizing or recognizing visual stimuli; may be unable to sustain or shift focus between objects or words; or be unable to sustain, shift, or divide attention within or between language modalities (e.g., vision and audition). These difficulties increase the cognitive load for all visual language activities and make it difficult to understand and remember when reading.

Effective assessment and treatment of acquired reading and writing disorders begins with the examination of both central and peripheral components of reading and writing. The clinician should also address both phonological working memory and visual working memory to improve memory for sequences of letters and words, which will support reading comprehension in the client with a peripheral reading disorder. The rehabilitative process should include consultation with occupational therapy and neuro-optometry whenever possible to identify signs of visual system function and implement vision rehabilitation measures when indicated. In Chapter 3, we will review formal tests that differentiate central and peripheral visual language impairments. Methods for adapting speech-language pathology assessment and treatment protocols to accommodate visual system dysfunction and support vision rehabilitation efforts in the brain-injured population will be discussed.

REFERENCES

Abelson, M. (2011). It's time to think about the blink. *Review of Ophthalmology*. Retrieved from https://www.reviewofophthalmology.com. Accessed on December 17, 2018.

Ajina, S. & Rees, G. (2011). Unconscious processing following visual cortex damage. *Advances in Clinical Neuroscience and Rehabilitation*, 11(3), 24-27.

Amalnath, S. D., Kumar, S., Deepanjoli, S., & Dutta, T. K. (2014). Balint syndrome. *Annals of Indian Academy of Neurology*, 17(1), 10-11.

Azouvi, P., Bartolomeo, P., Beis, J-M., Prennou, D., Pradat-Diehl, P. & Rousseax, M. (2006). A battery of tests for the quantitative assessment of unilateral neglect. *Restorative Neurology and Neuroscience, 24*, 273-385.

Baddeley, A. D. (2003). Working memory and language: An overview. *Journal of Communication Disorders, 36*, 189-208.

Baddeley, A. D. (2007). *Working memory, thought and action.* New York, NY: Oxford University Press.

Baddeley, A. D. (2012). Working memory: Theories, models and controversies. *Annual Review of Psychology, 63*, 1-29.

Baines, K., Martin, A., & McMartin Heeringa, H. (1999). *The Assessment of language-related functional activities.* Austin, TX: Pro-Ed.

Baker, G. E. (2000). Visual pathways, module 2, part 1 & 3. *Optometry Today.*

Barbato, M. & Addington, J. (2014). Binocular depth perception in individuals at clinical high risk for psychosis: No evidence of dysfunction. *Neuropsychology, 28*(3), 366-372.

Bauer, R. M. (2012). Agnosia. In: K. M. Heilman, & E. Valenstein (Eds.). *Clinical neuropsychology* (5th ed) (pp. 238-295). New York, NY: Oxford University Press.

Bayles, K. A., Kaszniak, A. W., & Tomoeda, C. K. (1987). Perception and attention in normal aging and dementia. In: K. A. Barles, & A. W. Kaszniak (eds.), *Communication and Cognition in Normal Aging and Dementia.* Austin, TX: Pro-Ed.

Beeson, P. M., Rewega, M. A., Vail, S., & Rapcsak, S. Z. (2000). Problem-solving approach to agraphia treatment: Interactive use of lexical and sublexical spelling routes. *Aphasiology, 14*(5-6), 551-565.

Behrmann, M., Shomstein, S. S., Black, S. E., & Barton, J. (2001). The eye movements of pure alexia patients during reading and nonreading tasks. *Neuropsychologia, 39*, 982-1002.

Behrmann, M., Black, S. E., McKeef, T. F., & Barton J. (2002). Oculographic analysis of word reading in hemispatial neglect. *Physiology and Behavior, 77*, 613-619.

Beis, J. M., Keller, C., Morin, N., Bartolomeo, P., Bernati, T., Chokron, S., ... Azouvi, P. (2004). French right spatial neglect after left hemisphere stroke: Qualitative and quantitative Study. *Neurology, 63*(9), 1600-1605.

Bertone, A., Bettinelli, L., & Faubert, J. (2007). The impact of blurred vision on cognitive assessment. *Journal of Clinical and Experimental Neuropsychology, 29*(5), 467-476.

Beschin, N., Cisari, C., Cubelli, R., & Della Sala, S. (2014). Prose reading in neglect. *Brain and Cognition, 84*, 69-75.

Bhatti, M.T., Schmalfuss, I. M., Williams, L., & Quisling, R. G. (2003). Peripheral third cranial nerve enhancement in multiple sclerosis. *American Journal of Neuroradiology, 24*, 1390-1395.

Bhatti, M. T., Eisenschenk, S., Roper, S., & Guy, J. R. (2006). Superior divisional third cranial nerve paresis. *Archives of Neurology, 63*, 771-776.

Black, S., Behrmann, M., Bass, K., & Hacker, P. (1989). Selective writing impairment: Beyond the allographic code. *Aphasiology, 3*, 265-277.

Bridge, H., Thomas, O., Jhabdi, S., & Cowey, A. (2008). Changes in connectivity after visual cortical brain damage underlie altered visual function. *Brain, 131*, 1433-1444.

Bristow, D., Frith, C., & Rees, G. (2005). Blinking suppresses the neural response to unchanging retinal stimulation. *Current Biology, 15*, 1296-1300.

Broca, P. P. (1861). Perde de la parole, ramollissement chronique et destruction partielle du lobe anterior gauche du cerveau [Loss of speech, chronic softening and partial destruction of the anterior left lobe of the brain]. *Bulletin de la Société Anthropologique, 12*, 235-238.

Brouwer, G. J., van Ee, R., & Schwarzbach, J. (2005). Activation in visual cortex correlates with the awareness of stereoscopic depth. *Journal of Neuroscience, 25*(45), 10403-10413.

Brussee T., van den Berg, T. J., van Nispen, R., & van Rens, G. H. (2017). Associations between spatial and temporal contrast sensitivity and reading. *Optometry and Vision Science, 94*(3), 329-338.

Buchel, C., Coull, J., & Friston, K. (1999). The predictive value of changes in effective connectivity for human learning. *Science, 283*, 1538-1541.

Buonomano, D. V. & Merzenich, M. M. (1998). Cortical plasticity: From synapses to maps. *Annual Reviews Neuroscience, 21*, 149-186.

Burr, D. (2005). Vision in the blink of an eye. *Current Biology, 15*(14), R554-R556. doi: 10.1016/j.cub.2005.07.007.

Burton, J. J., Press, D. Z., Keenan, J. P., & O'Connor, M. (2002). Lesions of the fusiform face area impair perception of facial configuration in prosopagnosia. *Neurology, 58*(1), 71-78.

Calautti, C. & Baron, J-C. (2003). Functional neuroimaging studies of motor recovery after stroke in adults. *Stroke, 34*, 1553-1566.

Calvert, G., Campbell, R., & Brammer, M. (2000). Evidence from functional magnetic resonance imaging of polymodal binding in the human heteromodal cortex. *Current Biology, 110*, 649-657.

Campion, J., Latto, R., & Smith, Y. M. (1983). Is blindsight an effect of scattered light, spared cortex, and near-threshold vision? *Behavioral and Brain Sciences, 6*, 423-486.

Caramazza, A. & Hillis, A. E. (1990). Spatial representation of words in the brain implied by studies of a unilateral neglect patient. *Nature, 346*, 267-269.

Caramazza, A., Miceli, G., Villa G., & Romani, C. (1987). The role of the graphemic buffer in spelling: Evidence from a case of acquired dysgraphia. *Cognition, 26*, 59-85.

Carter, A. R., Shulman, G. L., & Corbetta, M. (2012). Why use a connectivity-based approach to study stroke and recovery of function? *Neuroimage, 62*(4), 2271-2280.

Caselli, R. (2000). Visual syndromes as the presenting features of degenerative brain disease. *Seminars in Neurology, 20*(1), 139-144.

Ciuffreda, K. J. & Kapoor, N. (2007). Oculomotor dysfunctions, their remediation, and reading-related problems in mild traumatic brain injury. *Journal of Behavioral Optometry, 18*(3), 72-77.

Ciuffreda, K. J., Kapoor, N., Rutner, D., Suchoff, I. B., Han, M. E., & Craig, S. (2007). Occurrence of oculomotor dysfunction in acquired brain injury: A retrospective analysis. *Optometry, 78,* 155-161.

Ciuffreda, K. J., Rutner, D., Kapoor N., Suchoff, I. B., Craig, S., & Han, M. E. (2008). Vision therapy for oculomotor dysfunctions in acquired brain injury: A retrospective analysis. *Optometry, 79,* 18-22.

Cloutman, L., Gingis, L., Newhart, M., Davis, C., Heidler-Gary, J., Crinion, J., & Hillis, A. E. (2009). A neural network crucial for spelling. *Annals of Neurology, 66,* 249-253.

Corbetta, M., Kincade, J. M., Lewis, C., Snuder, A. Z., & Sapir, A. (2005). Neural basis and recovery of spatial attention deficits in spatial neglect. *Nature Neuroscience, 8,* 1603-1610.

Corbetta, M. & Shulman, G. (2011). Spatial neglect and attention networks. *Annual Review of Neuroscience, 34,* 569-599.

Cramer, S., Sur, M., Dobkin, B. H., O'Brien, C., Sanger, T. D., Trojanowski, J. Q., …Vinograd, S. (2011). Harnessing neuroplasticity for clinical applications. *Brain, 134*(6), 1591-1609.

Das, A. & Gilbert, C. D. (1995). Receptive field expansion in adult visual cortex is linked to dynamic changes in strength of cortical connections. *Journal of Neurophysiology, 74,* 779-792.

Davies, E. J., Coughlin, T., & Ellis, A. W. (1997). Peripheral dysgraphia with impaired processing of musical and other symbols. *Journal of Neurolinguistics, 10*(1), 11-17.

Davis, C. J. & Coltheart, M. (2002). Paying attention to reading errors in acquired dyslexia. *Trends in Cognitive Sciences, 6*(9), 359-361.

de Gelder, B. (2010). Uncanny sight in the blind. *Scientific American, 302*(5), 60-65.

de Rodrigues, J., de Fontoura, D., & de Salles, J. (2014). Acquired dysgraphia in adults following right or left hemisphere stroke. *Dementia & Neuropsychologia, 8*(3), 236-242.

Dehaene, S. (2009). *Reading in the brain: The science and evolution of a human invention.* New York, NY: Viking Penguin.

Dehaene, S. (2014). *Consciousness and the brain: Deciphering how the brain codes our thoughts.* New York, NY: Penguin Books.

Devinsky, O. & D'Esposito, M. (2004). *Neurology of cognitive and behavioral disorders.* New York, NY: Oxford University Press.

Dos Santos, N. & Andrade, S. (2012). Visual contrast sensitivity in patients with impairment of functional independence after stroke. *BMC Neurology, 12*(90), 1-7.

Edmans, J. & Lincoln, N. B. (1987). The frequency of perceptual deficits after stroke. *Clinical Rehabilitation, 1,* 273-281.

Emerson, M. J. & Miyake, A. (2003). The role of inner speech in task switching: A dual-task investigation. *Journal of Memory and Language, 48,* 148-168.

Epelbaum, S., Pinel, P., Gaillard, R., Delmaire, C., Perrin, M., DuPont, S., & Cohen, L. (2008). Pure alexia as a disconnection syndrome: New diffusion imaging evidence for an old concept. *Cortex, 44*(8), 962-974.

Evans, J. J., Heggs, A. J., Antoun, N., & Hodges, J. R. (1995). Progressive prosopagnosia associated with selective right temporal lobe atrophy. *Brain, 118*(1), 1-13.

Fahle, M. & Greenlee, M. (2003). *The neuropsychology of vision.* New York, NY: Oxford University Press.

Farah, M. J., Hammond, K. M., Levine, D. N., & Calvanio, R. (1988). Visual and spatial mental imagery: Dissociable systems of representation. *Cognitive Psychology, 20,* 213-218.

Farah, M. J. (2000). *The cognitive neuroscience of vision.* Malden, MA: Blackwell Publishing.

Farah, M. J. (2004). Visual form agnosia. In: *Visual agnosia* (2nd ed.). Cambridge, MA: MIT Press.

Fendrich, R., Wessinger, C. M., & Gazzinga, M. S. (1992). Residual vision in a scotoma: Implications for blindsight. *Science, New Series, 258*(5087), 1489-1491.

Fletcher, P., Buchel, C., Josephs, O., Friston, K., & Dolan, R. (1999). Learning-related neuronal responses in prefrontal cortex studied with functional neuroimaging. *Cerebral Cortex, 9,* 168-178.

Friedman, R. B. & Alexander, M. P. (1989). Written spelling agraphia. *Brain and Language, 36,* 503-517.

Garavan, H., Kelley, D., Rosen, A., Rao, S. M., & Stein, E. A. (2000). Practice-related functional activation changes in a working memory task. *Microscopic Research and Technique, 51,* 54-63.

Geva, S., Bennett, S., Warburton, E. A., & Patterson, K. (2011). Discrepancy between inner and overt speech: Implications for post-stroke aphasia and normal language processing. *Aphasiology, 25,* 323-343.

Gianutsos, R. (1997). Vision rehabilitation following acquired brain injury. In: M. Gentile (Ed.), *Functional visual behavior: A therapist's guide to evaluation and treatment options.* Bethesda, MD: American Occupational Therapy Association, Inc.

Gianutsos, R. & Matheson, P. (1987). The rehabilitation of visual perceptual disorders attributable to brain injury. In: M. Meier, A. Benton, & L. Diller (Eds.), *Neuropsychological rehabilitation.* London, UK: Churchill-Livingstone.

Giaschi, D., Jan, J., Young, S., Tata, M., Lyons, C., Good, W., & Wong, P. (2003). Conscious visual abilities in a patient with early bilateral occipital damage. *Developmental Medicine and Child Neurology, 45*(11), 772-781.

Gillen, G. (2009). *Cognitive and perceptual rehabilitation: Optimizing function.* St. Louis, MO: Mosby Elsevier.

Glisson, CC. (2014). Visual loss due to optic chiasm and retrochiasmal visual pathway lesions. *Continuum, 20*: 907-921.

Globe, L. I., Davis, P. H., Schoeberg, B. S., & Duvoisin, R. C. (1988). Prevalence and natural history of progressive supranuclear palsy. *Neurology, 38*(7), 1031-1034.

Goldman-Rakic, P. (1988). Topography of cognition: Parallel distributed networks in primate association cortex. *Annual Reviews Neuroscience, 11*, 137-156.

Golomb, J. & Kanwisher, N. (2011). Higher level visual cortex represents retinotopic, not spatiotopic, object location. *Cerebral Cortex, 12*, 2794-2810.

Gonzalez, F., Relova, J. L., Prieto, A., & Peleteiro, M. (2005). Evidence of temporo-occipital cortex involvement in stereoscopic vision in humans: A study with subdural electrode recordings. *Cerebral Cortex, 15*(1), 117-122.

Goodglass, H. & Kaplan, E. (1972). *Boston diagnostic aphasia examination.* Lutz, FL: Psychological Assessment Resources.

Goodglass H. & Weintraub, S. (2001). *Boston naming test.* Philadelphia, PA: Lippincott, Williams & Wilkins.

Green, W., Ciuffreda, K. J., Thiagarajan, P., Szymanowicz, D., Ludlam, D. P., & Kapoor, N. (2010a). Static and dynamic aspects of accommodation in mild traumatic brain injury: A review. *Optometry, 81*(3), 129-136.

Green, W., Ciuffreda, K. J., Thiagarajan, P., Szymanowicz, D., Ludlam, D. P., & Kapoor, N. (2010b). Accommodation in mild traumatic brain injury. *Journal of Rehabilitation Research and Development, 47*(3), 183-200.

Halligan, P. W., Fink, G. R., Marshall, J. C., & Vallar, G. (2003). Spatial cognition: Evidence from visual neglect. *Trends in Cognitive Neuroscience, 7*(3), 125-133.

Hand, C. J., O'Donnell, P. J., & Sereno, S.C. (2012). Word-initial letters influence fixation durations during fluent reading. Frontiers in Psychology. *Language Sciences, 3*(85), 1-19.

Heilman, K. M. & Valenstein, E. (2012). *Clinical neuropsychology* (5th ed) (pp. 238-295). New York, NY: Oxford University Press.

Heuninckx, S., Winderoth, N., & Swinnen, S. P. (2008). Systems neuroplasticity in the aging brain: Recruiting additional neural resources for successful motor performance in elderly persons. *The Journal of Neuroscience, 28*(1), 91-99.

Hickok, G. & Poeppel, D. (2004). Dorsal and ventral streams: A framework for understanding aspects of the functional anatomy of language. *Cognition, 92*, 67-99.

Hickok, G. and Poeppel, D. (2007). The cortical organization of speech processing. *Nature Reviews Neuroscience, 8*, 393-402.

Hillis, A. E., Newhart, M., Heidler, J., Barker, P. B., Herskovitz, E. H., & Degaonkar, M. (2005). Anatomy of spatial attention: Insights from perfusion imaging and hemispatial neglect in acute stroke. *The Journal of Neuroscience, 25*(12), 3161-3167.

Hillis, A. E. (2006). Rehabilitation of unilateral spatial neglect: New insights from magnetic resonance perfusion imaging. *Archives of Physical Medicine and Rehabilitation, 887*(12 Supplement 2), S43-S49.

Holland, M. & Tarlow, G. (1972). Blinking and mental load. *Psychological Representation, 31*(1), 119-127.

Hubel, D. H. (1995). The eye. In: *Eye, Brain and Vision.* New York, NY: WH Freeman and Company.

Humphreys, G. W. & Riddoch, M. J. (1995). Separate coding of space within and between perceptual objects: Evidence from unilateral visual neglect. *Cognitive Neuropsychology, 12*(3), 283-311.

Jackson, G. R. & Owsley, C. (2003). Visual dysfunction, neurodegenerative diseases, and aging. *Neurologic Clinics of North America, 21*, 709-729.

James, T. W., Culham, J., Humphrey, G. K., Milner, A. D., & Goodale, M. A. (2003). Ventral occipital lesions impair object recognition but not object-directed grasping: An fMRI study. *Brain, 126*(Pt 11), 2463-2475.

Kandel, E.R., Schwartz, J.H., & Jessel, T.M. (1995). Visual processing by the retina. In: *Essentials of neural science and behavior.* East Norwalk, CT: Appleton Lange.

Kanwisher, N., McDermott, J., & Chun, M. (1997). The fusiform face area: A module in human extrastriate cortex specialized for face perception. *Journal of Neuroscience, 17*, 4302-4311.

Kerkhoff, G. (2000). Neurovisual rehabilitation: Recent developments and future directions. *Journal of Neurology, Neurosurgery & Psychiatry, 68*, 691-706.

Kerkhoff, G. & Schenk, T. (2012). Rehabilitation of neglect: An update. *Neuropsychologia, 50*, 1072-1079.

Kertesz, A. (1982). *Western aphasia battery.* San Diego, CA: Harcourt Brace Jovanovich.

Kim, E. S. & Lemke, S. F. (2016) Behavioural and eye movement outcomes in response to text-based reading treatment for acquired alexia. *Neuropsychological Rehabilitation: An International Journal, 26* (1): 60-86.

Kim, E. S., Rapcsak, S. Z., Anderson, S., & Beeson, P. M. (2011). Multimodal alexia: Neuropsychological mechanisms and implications for treatment. *Neuropsychologia, 49*, 3551-3562.

Kim, E. S., Rising, K., Rapcsak, S. Z., & Beeson, P. M. (2015). Treatment for alexia with agraphia following left ventral occipito-temporal damage: Strengthening orthographic representations common to reading and spelling. *Journal of Speech, Language and Hearing Research, 58*, 1521-1537.

Kleim, J. A. & Jones, T. A. (2008). Principles of experience-dependent neural plasticity: Implications for rehabilitation after brain damage. *Journal of Speech, Language and Hearing Research, 51*(Suppl.), S225-S239.

Kleim, J. A., Bruneau, R., VandenBerg, P, MacDonald, E., Mulrooney, R., & Pocock, D. (2005). Motor cortex stimulation enhances motor recovery and reduces peri-infarct dysfunction following ischemic insult. *Neurological Research, 2*, 789-793.

Kleinman, J. T., Newhart, M., Davis, C., Heidler-Gary, J., Gottesman, R. F., & Hillis, A. E. (2007). Right hemispatial neglect: Frequency and characterization following acute left hemisphere stroke. *Brain and Cognition, 64*(1), 50-59.

Lambert, J., Giffard, B., Nore, F., de la Sayette V., Pasquier, F., & Eustache, F. (2007). Central and peripheral agraphia in Alzheimer's disease: From the case of Augustus D. to a cognitive neuropsychology approach. *Cortex, 43*(7), 935-951.

Lambon Ralph, M. A. & Ellis, A. W. (1997). 'Patters of Paralexia' revisited: Report of a case of visual dyslexia. *Cognitive Neuropsychology, 7*, 953-974.

LaPointe, L. & Horner, J. (2006). *The reading comprehension battery for aphasia-2*. Austin, TX: Pro-ed, Inc.

Laurent, L., Millot, J. L., Andrieu, P., Camos, V., Floccia, C., & Mathy, F. (2016). Inner speech sustains predictable task switching: Direct evidence in adults. *Journal of Cognitive Psychology, 28*, 585-592.

Leff, A. P., Scott, S. K., Crewes, H., Hodgson, T. L., Cowey, A., Howard D., & Wise, R. J. (2000). Impaired reading in patients with right hemianopia. *Annals of Neurology, 47*(2), 171-178.

Leff, A. P., Crewes, H., Plant, G. T., Scott, S. K., Kennard, C., & Wise, R. J. (2001). The functional anatomy of single-word reading in patients with hemianopic and pure alexia. *Brain, 124*, 510-521.

Leff, A. P. & Schofield, T. M. (2010). Rehabilitation of acquired alexia. In: J.H. Stone & M. Blouin (Eds.). *International Encyclopedia of Rehabilitation*. Buffalo, NY: University at Buffalo.

Leh, S., Johansen-Berg, H., & Ptito, A. (2006). Unconscious vision: New insights into the neuronal correlate of blindsight using diffusion tractography. *Brain, 129*(7), 1822-1832.

Levi, D. M. & Polat, U. (1996). Neural plasticity in adults with amblyopia. *Proceedings of the National Academy of Science, 93*, 6830-6834.

Lewis, J., Beauchamp, M., & DcYoc, E. (2000). A comparison of visual and auditory motion processing in human visual cortex. *Cerebral Cortex, 10*(9), 878-888.

Lissauer, H. (1890). Ein fall von seelenblindheit nebst einem Beitrag zur Theorie derselben [A case of visual agnosia with a contribution to theory]. *Archives Psychiatric, 21*, 222-270.

Livingstone, M. (2006). *Advances in brain research: Conversations with seven leading neuroscientists on timely topics in brain research*. News Office.

Lott, S. N., Carney, A. S., Glezer, L. S., & Friedman, R. B. (2010). Overt use of tactile-kinesthetic strategy shifts to covert processing in rehabilitation of letter-by-letter reading. *Aphasiology, 24*(11), 1424-1442.

Magrassi, L., Bongetta, D., Bianchini, S., Berardesca, M., & Arienta, C. (2010). Central and peripheral components of writing critically depend on a defined area of the dominant superior parietal gyrus. Brain Research, *134*, 145-154.

Mahncke, H., Bronstone, A., & Merzenich, M. M. (2006). Brain plasticity and functional losses in the aged: Scientific bases for a novel intervention. *Progress in Brain Research, 157*, 81-109.

Margolis, N. W. (2011). Evaluation and treatment of visual field loss and visual-spatial neglect. In: P. S. Suter, & L. H. Harvey (Eds.), *Vision Rehabilitation: Multidisciplinary care of the patient following brain injury*. Boca Raton, FL: CRC Press.

Marsh, F. & Hillis, A. (2008). Dissociation between egocentric and allocentric visuospatial and tactile neglect in acute stroke. *Cortex, 44*, 1215-1220.

McCandliss, B. D., Cohen, L., & Dehaene S. (2003). The visual word form area: Expertise for reading in the fusiform gyrus. *Trends in Cognitive Neuroscience, 7*(7), 293-299.

McConkie, G. W. & Rayner, K. (1976). Asymmetry of the perceptual span in reading. *Bulletin of Psychonomic Sociology, 8*, 365-368.

McIntosh, A. R. (2000). Towards a network theory of cognition. *Neural Networks, 3*, 861-870.

Medina, J., Kannan, V., Pawlak, M. A., Kleinman, J. T., Newhart, M., Davis, C., ... Hillis, A. E. (2009). Neural substrates of visuospatial processing in distinct reference frames: Evidence from unilateral spatial neglect. *Journal of Cognitive Neuroscience, 21*(11), 2073-2084.

Menichelli, A., Rapp, B., & Semenza, C. (2008). Allographic agraphia: A case study. *Cortex, 44*, 861-868.

Menichelli, A., Machetta, F., Zadini, A., & Semenza, C. (2012). Allographic agraphia for single letters. *Behavioural Neurology, 25*, 1-12.

Merriam, E. P. & Colby, C. L. (2005). Active vision in parietal and extrastriate cortex. *The Neuroscientist*. Retrieved from http://www.cnbc.cmu.edu/~ccolby/papers/MerriamColby2005.pdf

Merzenich, M. M., Jenkins, W. M., Johnston, P., Schreiner, C., Miller, S. L., & Tallal, P. (1996). Temporal processing deficits of language-learning impaired children ameliorated by training. *Science, 271*, 77-81.

Mesulam, M. (1990). Large-scale neurocognitive networks and distributed processing for attention, language and memory. *Annals of Neurology, 28*(5), 597-613.

Miller, L. J., Mittenberg, W., Carey, V. M., McMorrow, M. A., Kashner, T. E., & Weinstein, J. M. (1999). Asteropsis caused by traumatic brain injury. *Archives of Clinical Neuropsychology, 14*(6), 537-543.

Milner, A. D., Perrett, D. I., Johnston, R. S., Benson, P. J., Jordan, T. R., Heeley, D. W., ... Davidson, D.L. (1991). Perception and action in 'visual form agnosia'. *Brain, 114*, 405-428.

Milner, A. D. & Goodale, M. A. (2006). *The Visual brain in action* (2nd ed.). New York, NY: Oxford University Press.

Milner, A. D. & Goodale, M. A. (2008). Two visual systems reviewed. *Neuropsychologia, 46*, 774-785.

Mittenberg, W., Choi, E. J., & Apple, C. C. (2000). Stereoscopic visual impairment in vascular dementia. *Archives of Clinical Neuropsychology 15*(7), 561-569.

Moore, J. S. (1986). Recovery potentials following CNS lesions: A brief historical perspective in relation to modern research data on neuroplasticity. *Journal of Occupational Therapy, 40*(7), 459-463.

Moreno, D. R., Schiff, N. D., Giacino, J., Kalmar, K., & Hirsch, J. (2010). A network approach to assessing cognition in disorders of consciousness. *Neurology, 75*(21), 1871-1878.

Mort, D. & Kennard, C. (2000). Adult neuro-degenerative diseases and their neuro-ophthalmological features. *Optometry Today, 2*(Part 7), 33-37.

Munoz-Cespedes, J. M., Rios-Lago, M., & Maestu, F. (2005). Functional neuroimaging studies of cognitive recovery after acquired brain damage in adults. *Neuropsychological Review, 15*, 169-183.

Naeser, M. A. & Hayward, R. W. (1978). Lesion localization in aphasia with cranial computed tomography and the Boston Diagnostic Aphasia Exam. *Neurology, 28*(6), 545-551.

Newcombe, F. & Ratcliff, G. (1989). Disorders of visuospatial analysis. In: S. B. Filskov, & T. J. Boll (Eds.), *Handbook of Neuropsychology*. (pp. 335-356). Hoboken, NJ: John Wiley & Sons.

Nichelli, P., Venneri, A., Pentore, R., & Cubelli, R. (1993). Horizontal and vertical neglect dyslexia. *Brain and Language, 44*, 264-283.

Nichol, T. & Krauss, N. (2004). Speech-sound encoding: Physiological manifestations and behavioral ramifications. *Advances in Clinical Neurophysiology, 57*(Suppl.), 624-630.

Padula, W. V., Shapiro, J., & Jasin, P. (1988). Head injury causing post trauma vision syndrome. *New England Journal of Optometry, 41*(2), 16-20.

Papagno, C. (2002). Progressive impairment of constructional abilities: A visuospatial sketchpad deficit? *Neuropsychologia, 40*, 1858-1867.

Parton, A., Malhotra, P., & Husain, M. (2004). Hemispatial neglect. *Journal of Neurology, Neurosurgery & Psychiatry, 75*, 13-21.

Pelli, D.G., Palomares, M. & Majaj, N.J. (2004). Crowding is unlike ordinary masking: Distinguishing feature integration from detection. Journal of Vision, 4, 1136-1169.

Pelli, D.G., Tillman, K.A., Freeman, J., Su, M., Berger, T.D., & Majaj, N.J. (2007). Crowding and eccentricity determine reading rate. Journal of Vision, 7(2):20, 1-36.

Perenin, M-T. & Jeannerod, M. (1978). Visual function within the hemianopic field following early hemidecortication in man—I. Spatial localization. *Neuropsychologia, 16*, 1-13.

Petzinger, G. M., Fisher, B. E., McEwen, S., Beeler, J. A., Walsh, J. P., & Jakowec, M. W. (2013). Exercise-enhanced neuroplasticity targeting motor and cognitive circuitry in Parkinson's Disease. *Lancet Neurology, 12*(7), 716-726.

Pflugshaupt, T., Gutbrod, K., Wurtz, P., von Wartburg, R., Nyffelert, T., de Haan, B., ... Mueri, R. M. (2009). About the role of visual field defects in pure alexia. *Brain, 132*, 1907-1917.

Planton, S., Jucla, M., Roux, F-E., & Demonet, J-F. (2013). The "handwriting brain": A meta-analysis of neuroimaging studies of motor versus orthographic processes. *Cortex, 49*, 2772-2787.

Pöppel, E., Held, R., & Frost, D. (1973). Residual visual function after brain wounds involving the central visual pathways in man. *Nature, 243*, 295-296.

Possin, K. (2010). Visual spatial cognition in neurodegenerative disease. *Neurocase, 16*(6), 466-487.

Powell, J. M. & Torgerson, G. (2011). Evaluation and treatment of vision and motor dysfunction following acquired brain injury from occupational therapy and neuro-optometry perspectives. In: P. S. Suter, & L. H. Harvey (Eds.), *Vision rehabilitation: Multidisciplinary care of the patient following brain injury* (pp. 356-396). Boca Raton, FL: CRC Press.

Primativo, S., Arduiino, L. S., De Luca, M., Daini, R., & Martelli, M. (2013). Neglect dyslexia: A matter of "good looking". *Neuropsychologia, 51*, 2109-2119.

Pula, J. H. & Yuen, C. A. (2017). Eyes and stroke: the visual aspects of cerebrovascular disease. *Stroke and Vascular Neurology*; 2:e000079. doi: 10.1136/svn-2017-000079.

Purcell, J. J., Turkeltaub, P. E., Eden, G. F., & Rapp, B. (2011). Examining the central and peripheral processes of written word production through meta-analysis. *Frontiers of Psychology, 2*, 1-16.

Purcell, J. J., Napoliello, E. M., & Eden, G. F. (2011a). A combined fMRI study of typed spelling and reading. *NeuroImage, 55*, 750-762.

Raichle, M., Fiez, J., Videen, T., Macleod, A., Pardo, J., Fox, P., & Petersen, S. (1994). Practice-related changes in human brain functional anatomy during nonmotor learning. *Cerebral Cortex, 4*, 8-26.

Rapcsak, S. Z. & Beeson, P. M. (2002). Neuroanatomical correlates of spelling and writing. In: A.R. Hillis (Ed.). *The handbook of adult language disorders: Integrating cognitive neuropsychology, neurology and rehabilitation*. New York, NY: Psychology Press.

Rapp, B. (2002). Uncovering the cognitive architecture of spelling. In: A.R. Hillis (Ed.). *The handbook of adult language disorders: Integrating cognitive neuropsychology, neurology and rehabilitation*. New York, NY: Psychology Press.

Ratcliff, G. & Ross, J. E. (1981). Visual perception and perceptual disorder. *British Medical Journal, 17*(2), 181-186.

Rauschecker, J. (1998). Cortical processing of complex sounds. *Current Opinion in Neurology, 8*(4), 516-521.

Rauschecker, J. (1999). Auditory cortical plasticity: A comparison with other sensory systems. *Trends in Neuroscience,* *22*, 74-80.

Rauschecker, J. & Tian, B. (2000). Colloquium: Mechanisms and streams for processing of "what" and "where" in auditory cortex. *Proceedings of the National Academy of Sciences, 97*(22), 11800-11806.

Rayner, K. (1979). Eye guidance in reading: Fixation locations within words. Perception, *8*(1), 21-30.

Rayner, K. (1998). Eye movements and attention in reading, scene perception, and visual search. *The Quarterly Journal of Experimental Psychology, 62*(8), 1457-1506.

Rayner, K. (2009). Eye movements and attention in reading, scene perception, and visual search. *The Quarterly Journal of Experimental Psychology, 62*(8), 1457-1506.

Rayner, K., Castelhano, M., & Yang, J. (2009). Eye movements and the perceptual span in order and younger readers. *Psychology and Aging, 24*(3), 755-760.

Rayner, K., Slattery, T. J., & Belanger, N. N. (2010). Eye movements, the perceptual span and reading speed. *Psychonomic Bulletin and Review, 17*(6), 834-839.

Reinhart, S., Schindler, I., & Kerkhoff, G. (2011). Optokinetic stimulation affects word omissions but not stimulus-centered reading errors in paragraph reading in neglect dyslexia. *Neuropsychologia, 49*, 2728-2735.

Rizzo, M. & Vecera, S. P. (2002). Psychoanatomical substrates of Balint's syndrome. *Journal of Neurology, Neurosurgery & Psychiatry, 72*(12), 162-178.

Ro, T. & Rafal, R. (2006). Visual restoration in cortical blindness: Insights from natural and TMS-induced blindsight. *Neuropsychological Rehabilitation, 16*(4), 377-396.

Ross, J. & Ma-Wyatt, A. (2004). Saccades actively maintain perceptual continuity. Nature Neuroscience, *7*(1), 65-69.

Rowe, F. (2011). Prevalence of ocular motor cranial nerve palsy and associations following stroke. *Eye (Low Vision), 25*(7), 881-887.

Sahraie, A., Trevethan, C. T., Weiskrantz, L., Olson, J., MacLeod, M. J., Murray, A. D., … Coleman, R. (2003). Spatial channels of visual processing in cortical blindness. *European Journal of Neuroscience, 18*(5), 1189-1196.

Saj, A., Verdon, V., Vocat, R., & Vuilleumier, P. (2012). Letter to the editor: The anatomy underlying acute versus chronic spatial neglect' also depends on clinical tests. *Brain, 135*, 1-5/e207.

Sakai, K., Hikoski, O., Miyauchi, S., Takino, R., Sasaki, Y., & Putz, B. (1998). Transition of brain activation from frontal to parietal areas in visuomotor sequence learning. *Neuroscience, 18*, 1827-1840.

Sanet, R. B. & Press, L. J. (2011). Spatial vision. In: P. S. Suter, & L. H. Harvey (Eds.), *Vision rehabilitation: Multidisciplinary care of the patient following brain injury* (pp. 77-151). Boca Raton, FL: CRC Press.

Saur, D., Kerher, B. W., Schrell, S., Kammerer, D., Kellmeyer, P., Vry, M-S., … Weiller, C. (2008). Ventral and dorsal pathways for language. *Proceedings of the National Academy of Sciences, 105*, 18035-18040.

Schaadt, A., Brandt, S. A., Kraft, A., & Kerkhoff, G. (2015). Holmes and Horrax (1919) revisited: Impaired binocular fusion as a cause of "flat vision" after right parietal brain damage—a case study. *Neuropsychologia, 69*, 31-8.

Schuett, S., Heywood, C. A., Kentridge, R.W., & Zihl, J. (2008) The significance of visual information processing in reading: Insights from hemianopic dyslexia. *Neuropsychologia, 46*, 2495-2462.

Scialfa, C., Line, D., & Lyman, B. (1987). Age differences in target identification as a function of retinal location and noise level: Examination of the useful field of view. *Psychology and Aging, 2*(1), 14-19.

Sims, P., Fletcher, J., Bergman, E., Breier, J., Foorman, B., Castillo, E., … Papanicolaou, A. C. (2002). Dyslexia-specific brain activation profile becomes normal following successful remedial training. *Neurology, 58*(2), 1203-1213.

Sonty, S., Mesulam, M-M., Weintraub, S., Johnson, N. A., Parrish, T. B., & Gitelman, D. R. (2007). Altered effective connectivity within the language network in Primary Progressive Aphasia. *The Journal of Neuroscience, 27*(6), 1334-1345.

Stone, S. P., Halligan, P. W., Wilson, B., Greenwood, R.J., & Marshall, J. C. (1991). Performance of age-matched controls on a battery of visuo-spatial neglect tests. *Journal of Neurology, Neurosurgery, and Psychiatry, 54*, 341-344.

Suter, P. S. (2004). Rehabilitation and management of visual dysfunction following traumatic brain injury. In: M. Ashley (Ed.), *Traumatic Brain Injury Rehabilitative Treatment and Case Management.* Boca Raton, FL: CRC Press LLC.

Suter, P. S. & Margolis, N. (2005). Managing visual field defects following brain injury. *Brain Injury/Professional, 2*, 26-28.

Szwed, M., Ventura, P., Querido, L., Cohen, L., & Dehaene, S. (2012). Reading acquisition enhances an early visual process of contour integration. *Developmental Science, 15*(1), 139-149.

Tainturier, M. J., & Rapp, B. C. (2004). Complex graphemes as functional spelling units: Evidence from acquired dysgraphia. *Neurocase, 10*(2), 122-131.

Temple, E., Deutsch, G., Poldrack, R., Miller, S., Talla, P., Mersenich, M.M., & Gabrieli, J.D. (2003). Neural deficits in children with dyslexia ameliorated by behavioral remediation: Evidence from fMRI. *Proceedings of the National Academy of Sciences, 100*, 2860-2865.

Thiagarajan, P., Ciuffreda, K. J., & Ludlam, D. P. (2011). Vergence dysfunction in mild traumatic brain injury (mTBI). *Ophthalmic & Physiological Optics, 31*, 456-48.

Thompson, C. & den Ouden, D.-B. (2008). Neuroimaging and recovery of language n aphasia. *Current Neurology and Neuroscience Reports, 8*, 475-483.

Tong, R. (2003). Primary visual cortex and visual awareness. *Nature Review Neuroscience, 4*(3), 219-229.

Trauzetti-Klosinski, S. & Reinhard, J. (1998). The vertical field border in hemianopia and its significance for fixation and reading. *Investigative Ophthalmology & Vision Science, 29*, 2177-2186.

Tse, P., Baumgartner, F., & Greenlee, M. (2010). Event-related functional MRI of cortical activity evoked by microsaccades, small visual-guided saccades, and eyeblinks in human visual cortex. *Neuroimage, 49*(1), 805-816.

Ullrich, L. & Roeltgen, D. P. (2012). Agraphia. In: K. M. Heilman, & D. Valenstein (Eds.), *Clinical Neuropsychology* (5th Ed.). New York, NY: Oxford University Press.

Ungerleider, L. G. & Mishkin, M. (1982). Two cortical visual systems. In: D. J. Ingle (Ed.), *Analysis of Visual Behavior* (pp. 549-586). Cambridge, MA: MIT Press.

Uzzell, B. P., Dolinskas, C. A., & Langfit, T. W. (1988). Visual field defects in relation to head injury severity: A neuropsychological study. *Archives of Neurology, 45*(4), 420-424.

Vallar, G. (2007). Spatial neglect, Balint-Holmes' and Gerstmann's syndrome and other spatial disorders. *CNS Spectrums, 12*(7), 527-536.

Vallar, G., Burani, C., & Arduino, L. S. (2010). Neglect dyslexia: A review of the neuropsychological literature. *Experimental Brain Research, 206*, 219-235.

Verdon, V., Schwartz, S., Lorblad, K. O., Hauert, C. A., & Vuilleumier, P. (2010). Neuroanatomy of hemispatial neglect and its functional components: A study using voxel-based lesion-symptom mapping. *Brain, 133*, 880-894.

Weiskrantz, L., Warrington, E., Sanders, M. D., & Marshall, J. (1974). Visual capacity in hemianopic field following a restricted occipital ablation. *Brain, 97*, 709-728.

Wheatstone, C. (1838). Contributions to the physiology of vision. Part the first on some remarkable and hitherto unobserved phenomena of binocular vision. *Philosophical Transactions of the Royal Society of London: Biological Sciences, 2*, 371-393.

White, S. J., Johnson, R. L., Liversedge, S. P. & Rayner, K. (2008). Eye movements when reading transposed text: The importance of word-beginning letters. *Journal of Experimental Psychology: Human Perception and Performance, 34*(5), 1261-1276.

Wolf, M. (2007). *Proust and the squid: The story and science of the reading brain.* New York, NY: HarperCollins Publishers.

Woodhead, Z.V.J., Ong, Y.-H., & Leff, A.P. (2015). Web-based therapy for hemianopic alexia is syndrome-specific. BMJ Innovations, 1:88-95.

Woodhead, Z. V., Penny W., Barnes, G. R., Crewes, H., Wise, R. J., Price C. J. & Leff, A. P. (2013). Reading therapy strengthens top-down connectivity inpatients with pure alexia. *Brain, 136*, 2579-2591.

Zeki, S. & Ffytche, D. H. (1998). The Riddoch syndrome: Insights into the neurobiology of conscious vision. *Brain, 121*, 25-45.

Zihl, J. (1995). Visual scanning behavior in clients with homonymous hemianopia. *Neuropsychologia, 33*, 287-303.

Zihl, J. (2000a). Localized CNS lesions and their effect on visual function. *Optometry Today, 2*(11), 33-39.

Zihl, J. (2000b). *Neuropsychological rehabilitation.* London, UK: Psychological Press Ltd.

Zihl, J. (2000c). *Rehabilitation of Visual Disorders after Brain Injury* (p. 75). Psychology Press, Ltd. East Sussex, UK.

TEST BANK

1. When we read, words to the right of the fixation point are viewed with the _____ in order to plan the next rightward eye movement. (Select 1)
   a. peripheral retina
   b. central retina
   c. parafoveal retina
   d. bipolar retina

2. Normal aging effects on the visual system include: (Select all that apply)
   a. reduced contrast sensitivity
   b. reduced visual processing speed
   c. decline in visual search ability
   d. reduction in the Useful Field of View

3. Vision specialists who typically assess and treat visual motor and visual sensory deficits directly following brain injury and stroke include: (Select all that apply)
   a. ophthalmologists
   b. occupational therapists
   c. speech language pathologists
   d. behavioral or neurooptometrists

4. The eye movements that serve object recognition, reading and writing include: (Select 1)
   a. contrast sensitivity, spatial orientation, fixation, and retinotopic organization
   b. peripheral vision, accommodation, spatial orientation, and fixation
   c. fixation, saccades, vergence, and accommodation
   d. contrast sensitivity, saccades, retinotopic organization and fixation

5. Two types of visual motor disorders are characteristic of bilateral occipitoparietal lesions. _____ affects motor planning and eye-hand coordination when reaching for objects such as a pencil or word cards, while _____ affects the ability to gaze shift toward a new target outside the central retinal field. (Select 1)
   a. optic ataxia, oculomotor apraxia
   b. verbal apraxia, optic ataxia
   c. oculomotor apraxia, optic ataxia
   d. hemianopia, hemispatial neglect

6. _____ is a visual sensory impairment that prevents the reader from seeing whole words and interferes with the guidance of eye movements for reading. (Select 1)
   a. peripheral retinal field loss
   b. parafoveal field loss
   c. upper visual field loss
   d. contrast sensitivity

7. Subjects who have experienced a left hemisphere stroke may demonstrate right hemispatial neglect.

     ___ True

     ___ False

8. _____ affects reading and writing when it results in the inability to recognize number, letter and word forms. (Select 1)

    a. optic ataxia

    b. visual agnosia

    c. visual motor impairment

    d. gaze apraxia

9. Readers will use the "letter-by-letter" reading strategy when they: (Select 1)

    a. have difficulty remembering what they just read

    b. have difficulty matching sounds with letters

    c. have hemispatial neglect

    d. have difficulty recognizing letter and word forms due to visual agnosia

10. A referral to occupational therapy for visual system testing should be initiated: (Select all that apply)

    a. when the client forgets to bring her glasses to speech therapy

    b. when error patterns on reading and writing tests/exercises show signs of visual system dysfunction (e.g. hemispatial neglect, letter duplication errors, writing uphill or downhill)

    c. when a client complains of visual changes post stroke or brain injury

    d. when reading is impaired due to receptive aphasia

3

Assessment and Treatment of Acquired Peripheral Reading and Writing Disorders

The assessment of visual language function is particularly complex because of the variety of reading and writing disorders found in the neurological population. Peripheral reading and writing disorders are the result of lesions that occur along a cortical network called the *visual word form system* (Vinckier et al., 2007) that extends in a posterior-to-anterior course from the occipital to temporal cortex ending in the fusiform gyrus, the *visual word form area*, in the left temporal lobe. Along this ventral visual pathway, visual line segments are bound to form letter strings and ultimately abstract word forms (Vinckier et al., 2007; Wilson et al., 2013), which are then associated with the lexical, phonological and semantic processes of central language function. Peripheral language disorders can also result from brainstem and subcortical lesions, or lesions of the frontal eye fields that impair eye movements for reading. The associated visual-motor and visual-sensory impairments are characterized by a range of symptoms. Some of these symptoms are obvious such as double vision or blurring, while others such as visual field loss are more covert (Kinsbourne & Warrington 1962; Gianutsos, 1997). It is common practice for physicians to wait six months before referring patients to neuro-optometry or ophthalmology, waiting for visual system changes to stabilize (Powell & Torgerson, 2011). Some brain-injured clients complete rehabilitation programs and still report that their vision is "not right" or that they are not able to read. Therefore, all persons who have experienced a neurological event such as stroke, brain injury, or tumor resection, should be tested for visual sensory and motor impairments (Teasell, Salter, Cotoi, Brar, & Donais, 2016; VA/DoD, 2009; 2010). Those clients who have recently visited their eye doctor may report 20/20 corrected vision. It is important to remember that this is a description of visual acuity and does not reflect a full assessment of visual motor or sensory function.

Addressing practitioners in the fields of optometry, ophthalmology, and occupational therapy, Powell and Torgerson (2011) report that some clients appear to have plateaued in their recovery due to undiagnosed visual system impairments. The authors state that the ongoing development of theories and discoveries relating to vision "… allows us, as clinicians and scientists, to begin devising more creative and effective treatments based on a more sophisticated and integrated view of visual and visual-motor systems." As speech-language pathologists we ought to familiarize ourselves with the signs and symptoms of visual motor and sensory system dysfunction, regularly

McMartin Heeringa, H. *The Visual Brain and Peripheral Reading and Writing Disorders: A Guide to Visual System Dysfunction for Speech–Language Pathologists*. (pp. 51-76).

	TABLE 3-1	
A COMPARISON OF ERRORS ATTRIBUTABLE TO MOTOR SPEECH AND CENTRAL LANGUAGE DYSFUNCTION VERSUS VISUAL SYSTEM DYSFUNCTION ON THE ASSESSMENT OF LANGUAGE-RELATED FUNCTIONAL ACTIVITIES		
ERROR TYPE	MOTOR SPEECH OR CENTRAL LANGUAGE ERRORS	VISUAL SYSTEM DYSFUNCTION OR VISION-RELATED ERRORS
Telling Time	• Reading the numbers that the clock hands point to instead of stating the time in hours and minutes (ie., reading "10 minutes to 4" as "four-one-zero") • Verbal paraphasic errors (e.g., saying "six" for "nine"); may make multiple attempts to self-correct • Perseveration on verbal responses	• Left field cut or left neglect (e.g., 3:50 is interpreted as 4 o'clock, as the client only sees the hour hand on 4
Counting Coins	• Substitution of one coin word ("nickel") for another ("quarter") • Count by 5s when they intend to count by 10s • Misinterpretation of question stimuli • Verbal perseveration	• Counting some of the coins, while neglecting others to the left of midline • Complaints of inability to differentiate between real coins and doubles; client may reach out to touch coins and then report that they have disappeared • Staring behavior • Postural changes
		(continued)

consult with occupational therapy or behavioral neuro-optometry when visual impairments are reported or suspected, and adapt our treatment methods to support vision rehabilitation efforts. A first step is to consult with occupational therapy regarding a client's visual history and results of the occupational therapy functional visual assessment. This typically includes measures of acuity, visual fields, visual motor function, visual attention, and scanning behavior (Cate & Richards, 2000; Gianutsos, 1997). Measures of near-point-of-convergence, useful field of view (UFOV), visual span, and contrast sensitivity are also important to the reading process (Cooper & Jamal, 2012; Dusek, Pierscionek, & McClelland, 2011; Jackson & Owsley, 2003; Rayner, Slattery, & Belanger, 2010;).

VISUAL LANGUAGE ASSESSMENT

When taking a client's history, the speech-language pathologist should ask about any activities a client may have curtailed such as reading, writing, or managing personal finances, and about any

	TABLE 3-1 (CONTINUED)	

A COMPARISON OF ERRORS ATTRIBUTABLE TO MOTOR SPEECH AND CENTRAL LANGUAGE DYSFUNCTION VERSUS VISUAL SYSTEM DYSFUNCTION ON THE ASSESSMENT OF LANGUAGE-RELATED FUNCTIONAL ACTIVITIES

ERROR TYPE	MOTOR SPEECH OR CENTRAL LANGUAGE ERRORS	VISUAL SYSTEM DYSFUNCTION OR VISION-RELATED ERRORS
Copying an Address	• Substitution of phonetically similar or semantically related words • Substitution of number words for numerals • Writing home address that is outdated, recognizing the error, and then duplicating the error	• Letter, number, or word omissions or duplications • Substitution of visually similar words • Letter/number sequence reversals • Letters and numbers from one line are incorporated into the line above or below • Writing uphill or downhill • Making many false starts; begins to write but cannot decide how to proceed • Word omissions in either visual field
Solving Daily Math Problems	• Reading aloud without comprehension • Errors in oral reading mislead client and take him or her off task • Perseveration on answers to previous question(s)	• Misreads $120.00 as $12.00 or $1200.00 • Fails to line up numbers in columns when writing out subtraction problem, which leads to mathematical errors • Mental math is better than calculating with paper and pencil

Source: Baines, K., Martin, A., & McMartin Heeringa, H. (1999). *Assessment of Language-Related Functional Activities.* Austin, TX: Pro-ed.

episodes of blurring or double vision. Clients who have experienced stroke, brain injury, tumor resection, or progressive neurological disease may not be aware of changes in their vision or visual language function (Townend et al., 2007; Margolis, 2011). They may report "I used to like to read a lot and watch TV, but now it doesn't interest me." Others report visual fatigue, headache, pressure at the temples or behind the eyes when reading, slow reading, or that visual stimuli are blurry, foggy, or dark (Kerkhoff, 2000; Zihl, 2000). Asking "What happens when you read?" will often elicit important details.

Whenever possible, language testing should be carried out with the client wearing his or her own reading glasses. Over-the-counter reading glasses in various strengths are useful when a client's own prescription glasses are not at hand. Sanet and Press (2011) report that clients with lesions in the dorsal visual pathway may no longer tolerate their progressive lenses. Presenting visual language stimuli at an angle (e.g., atop a binder or table-top easel) rather than flat on the table helps to reduce glare from direct light sources. Some clients reflexively place a hand above or alongside one eye or pull a baseball cap down over their forehead even in a dimly lit room. Dimming the lights or alternately covering one eye and then the other may help clients identify picture or word stimuli. Consultation with occupational therapy regarding the use of temporary eye patching may be beneficial.

Acquired reading and writing disorders are heterogenous (Greene, 2005; Leff et al., 2001). Effective treatment depends upon careful assessment of error patterns and identification of the specific type of reading or writing disorder demonstrated by each individual (e.g., aphasia, a central language disorder vs peripheral reading disorders [e.g., neglect dyslexia, alexia without agraphia, allographic agraphia]). Central reading and writing disorders are characterized by difficulty mapping from letters to sounds and mapping orthographic word forms to semantic representations. Peripheral reading disorders may be characterized by difficulty recognizing and naming letters, recognizing visual word forms, locating letters and words in relation to one another, sustaining focus, or scanning to read. Some clients will present with symptoms of both central and peripheral language impairments (Table 3-1). It may be necessary to administer portions of several language tests to fully evaluate reading and writing abilities. A sample of formal tests is listed in Appendix A and reviewed in the following paragraphs.

Arizona Battery for Reading and Spelling

The Arizona Battery for Reading and Spelling (ABRS) was developed by Pelagie Beeson and Kindle Rising as part of the Arizona Aphasia Project (American Speech-Language-Hearing Association [ASHA], 2011; Beeson & Rising, 2010). The ABRS is based on a *dual-route model* of written language processing (Beeson et al., 2008). According to this model the ability to spell irregular words (i.e., with irregular sound-letter correspondence) predicts the ability to retrieve whole words from the orthographic output lexicon (i.e., long-term memory for words). The ability to spell nonwords (i.e., pronounceable, made-up words) predicts non-lexical processing (i.e., the ability to use sound-letter conversion for written spelling). A sound-letter conversion deficit may be due to impairment in phonological processing or in the ability to process visual letter forms (see LaPointe & Horner, 2006). The ABRS measures oral reading as well as oral and written spelling of high- and low-frequency words and nonwords. Careful observation of response patterns may also reveal deficits in working memory for oral and written spelling, or a letter-sound conversion deficit in reading. Adult norms are included. Although this is not a timed test, it is useful to measure response latency during testing (Leff & Starrfelt, 2014) because a client may use letter-by-letter (LBL) reading to read or spell and decode words so slowly that he or she cannot recall a sequence of sounds or letters long enough to write the word down. The very slow decoding of words may suggest a *central visual pathway* deficit that can contribute to a peripheral reading or writing disorder. To download a copy of the ABRS, go to http://aphasia.arizona.edu.Aphasia_Research_Project/ For-Professionals.html

Reading Comprehension Battery for Aphasia-2

The Reading Comprehension Battery for Aphasia-2 Standard Battery (RCBA-2) (LaPointe & Horner, 2006) is a test of central language and silent reading comprehension. However, oral reading of paragraph stimuli can demonstrate error patterns associated with visual sensory or motor impairment involving one or both visual fields. For example, a right visual field deficit, or *viewer-centered neglect*, of the right visual field is suspected when the reader stops reading sentences aloud at midline or makes more oral reading errors to the right of midline (see Table 2-1). Conversely, when words are omitted only to the left of midline, a *viewer-centered neglect* of the left visual field is suspected. Repeated selection of response C on subtests I, II, III or VI of the RCBA-2 may indicate inattention to the left field, left hemianopia, or impaired gaze shifting toward the left. Whole word omissions or the substitution of visually-similar words (i.e., words that share the first three to four letters) across the entire visual field suggests *stimulus-centered neglect*. When oral reading illustrates a halting scan pattern with stops and starts, a visual motor impairment or scanning deficit is suspected. Some clients jump up or down a line or use a finger to block out the previous word to help them guide their eye movements for reading. They may also complain that words run together. These reading behaviors indicate the need for a formal, functional vision assessment. The reading assessment may be expanded with the RCBA-2 Supplemental Battery (Lapointe & Horner, 2006), which measures peripheral, or bottom-up, language skills including letter naming, letter recognition, and letter discrimination; central language functions including lexical decision making (i.e., discriminating real words from nonwords); and oral reading of single words and sentences. Careful examination of error patterns will help the speech-language pathologist differentiate a central from a peripheral reading disorder.

Visual field deficits and inattention are frequently associated with right hemisphere stroke and traumatic brain injury. Clients are assumed to be less vulnerable to visual system dysfunction following left hemisphere stroke (Beis et al., 2004; Greene, 2005) and are less likely to report changes in vision when expressive language deficits are present. However, they too may experience visual sensory or motor impairment. A study of eye movement patterns in left hemisphere stroke revealed that clients with Wernicke's aphasia make smaller, more frequent saccades, whereas, clients with Broca's aphasia demonstrated longer fixation times (Klingelhofer & Conrad, 1984). Another study found that clients with hemispatial neglect made fewer omission errors in both hemifields when scanning across rows of items vs items that are presented randomly (Weintraub & Mesulam, 1988). This may explain why clients with visual system dysfunction make more errors on the RCBA-2 subtest IV: functional reading, where the layout of each subtest item varies considerably, compared with subtest VII: paragraph-picture matching, where each item is presented in paragraph form (author observation). The following comments by a client with left hemisphere stroke and aphasia during administration of the RCBA-2 Standard Battery suggest a right visual field deficit: "It's warm over here (points to the left half of the paragraph she was reading), but when I get over here it's cold" (points to the right half of the paragraph). When error patterns suggest visual system dysfunction it is important to consult an occupational therapist or a behavioral neurooptometrist regarding a functional vision assessment.

Neuropsychological studies of acquired visual spatial impairment, including hemispatial neglect, generally rely on a standard test battery of paper-and-pencil tasks such as the Bells test (Gathercole, Gauthier, Dehaut, & Joanette, 1989), figure copying (Ogden, 1985), gap detection (Ota et al., 2001), and line bisection or clock drawing (Spreen & Strauss, 1998). However, reading assessments that include page-length passages in both one- and two-column format (i.e., newspaper format), and word-, phrase-, and sentence-length copying tasks are more sensitive to hemispatial neglect than traditional paper and pencil tests alone (Beschin, Cisari, Cubelli, & Della Sala, 2014; Edmans & Lincoln, 1987; Kleinman et al., 2007). Figure 3-1 illustrates an informal test for higher-functioning clients who may exhibit subtle signs of viewer-centered left hemispatial neglect but score high on formal reading tests (McMartin Heeringa, 2002). Hemispatial neglect may present in mobility testing and activities of daily living, but not in formal language testing. The converse is also possible.

Psycholinguistic Assessment of Language Processing Abilities

The psycholinguistic assessments of language processing abilities (PALPA; Kay, Lesser, & Coltheart, 1992; Kay et al., 1996) tests both central and peripheral reading and writing abilities. This test has been used by clinicians and in psycholinguistic research since 1992 (Bate, Kay, Code, Haslam, & Hollowell, 2010). In addition to measures of phonological processing, the 60 subtests of the psycholinguistic assessments of language processing abilities include separate measures of visual-orthographic processing (e.g., detecting mirror-reversed letters, matching upper- to lowercase letters), orthographic knowledge (i.e., converting lowercase letters to uppercase letters),

PRETEST: SECTION 7

INSTRUCTIONS: "Starting at the right margin, subtract '1' from the first number and write the answer on the line below it. Subtract '2' from the second number and write the answer on the line below it. Continue scanning right to left, subtracting '1' and '2' in alternating fashion until you reach the last number in each row at the left." Do the practice row first. (Clinician provides feedback after practice row). "It may help to say each number (1 or 2) aloud as you subtract it." The clinician may want to time each row to identify slower processing over time.

PRACTICE: 5   3   4   7   9   6   4   5   8   7

___ ___ ___ ___ ___ ___ ___ ___ ___ ___

6   3   9   7   8   5   6   3   7   4   9   5

___ ___ ___ ___ ___ ___ ___ ___ ___ ___ ___ ___

7   9   3   8   4   7   5   6   4   8   5   3

___ ___ ___ ___ ___ ___ ___ ___ ___ ___ ___ ___

4   3   5   2   6   3   9   8   5   6   4   7

___ ___ ___ ___ ___ ___ ___ ___ ___ ___ ___ ___

3   7   5   9   4   8   6   3   7   9   5   6

___ ___ ___ ___ ___ ___ ___ ___ ___ ___ ___ ___

8   4   5   6   3   9   7   4   8   3   6   5

___ ___ ___ ___ ___ ___ ___ ___ ___ ___ ___ ___

A Manual for the Treatment (Acquired Reading and Writing Disorders)

Figure 3-1. Informal test of hemispatial inattention. (McMartin Heeringa, H. [2002]. *A manual for the treatment of acquired reading and writing disorders.* Ann Arbor, Michigan: SLP Pathways.)

writing letter shapes, and letter naming. Performance on these peripheral language subtests is influenced by lexical variables such as word frequency, word imageability (i.e., ease with which one can perceive a word's meaning through association of the word with sensory properties such as color and shape; Paivio, 1986), and word length (Behrmann, Shomstein, Black, & Barton, 2001). These lexical variables may be selectively impaired following stroke (Menichelli, Rapp, & Semenza, 2008; Sinanović, Mrkonjić, Vidović, & Imamović, 2011). Additional testing might include writing or typing to dictation, written sentence formulation and written picture description, which engage both central and peripheral writing processes (Kim, Rapcsak, Anderson, & Beeson, 2011; Purcell, Turkeltaub, Eden, & Rapp, 2011).

Visagraph III Eye-Tracking System

The Visagraph III eye-tracking system (Bernell) provides objective, computer-based measures of visual motor function as they relate to reading comprehension and silent reading fluency (Tannen & Ciuffreda, 2007; Taylor, 2000). The Visagraph infrared goggles measure how well the eyes are working together as the client reads 100-word passages at various grade levels. Objective measures include the number of fixations; regressions (i.e., backward eye movements to reread a word or phrase); the duration of fixation in milliseconds; the span of recognition/UFOV (i.e. the number of words or objects recognized in a single fixation); and reading rate in words per minute. Norms are based on decades of research in eye movement patterns for reading. The Visagraph system is available to neurooptometrists, occupational therapists, educators, and speech-language pathologists at www.bernell.com/product. Objective measures such as those provided by the Visagraph III can be used to document the effectiveness of specific reading and writing treatment protocols.

Assessment of Language-Related Functional Activities

Tests that require a simple pointing response (e.g., the RCBA-2 Standard Battery [LaPointe & Horner, 2006]) are not sensitive enough to reveal underlying visual system deficits in some higher functioning clients. The Assessment of Language-Related Functional Activities (ALFA) (Baines, Martin, & McMartin Heeringa, 1999) provides objective measures of cognitive-communicative function in everyday language activities. The 10 ALFA subtests challenge clients to listen and read at the same time; count and manipulate bills and coins; copy an address exactly as presented; write a check; add and subtract numbers in columns; and write phone messages to dictation. These everyday language activities often reveal subtle signs of vision-related language dysfunction. Table 3-1 compares errors consistent with central language impairment to those that suggest visual sensory and motor impairment on the first four subtests of the ALFA. Clients with both central language deficits and visual system dysfunction will show a combination of these error patterns (author observation).

During administration of the ALFA some clients complain of blurring or double vision; difficulty with visual spatial relationships (e.g., copy letters out of sequence, write up- or downhill); or show signs of hemispatial neglect not evident on other language testing. Other clients add or subtract dollars and cents in their head, but are unable to sort and count bills and coins manually due to deficits in form recognition, visual attention, visual sensory function, visual spatial organization, or oculomotor function. Errors may include counting some coins while neglecting others to the left or right of midline. In cases of diplopia the client may report difficulty differentiating real coins from doubles. In cases of simultanagnosia, the client is only able to focus on one coin at a time and the coins seem to disappear and then reappear causing confusion. Postural changes, response delays, repeated loss of focus, impaired working memory, and staring behavior may also be noted.

After completing the cognitive-communicative evaluation, the speech-language pathologist should consult with occupational therapy to review any signs or symptoms of visual system dysfunction. At this point neuro-optometric consultation may be needed. Ophthalmologists are medical doctors who specialize in eye diseases and typically do not provide vision therapy. Behavioral neurooptometrists who provide rehabilitation services may have passed examinations administered by the American Academy of Optometry and the College of Optometrists in Vision Development (Scheiman, 2011). Vision rehabilitation methods include exercises, prisms, and compensation techniques for low vision. Helpful resources include the College of Optometrists in Vision Development at covd.org; and The Neuro-Optometric Rehabilitation Association, International at https://noravisionrehab.org, which provides a list of neurooptometrists by state. The reader may also wish to consult The American Academy of Optometry. Some clients report having been told by an ophthalmologist or optometrist that their corrected vision is fine despite their persistent visual symptoms. Vision testing that does not include measures of visual sensory function (e.g., visual fields, binocular function, contrast sensitivity, visual span, form recognition, depth perception, spatial perception) will overlook visual impairments in the brain-injured population. Visual system dysfunction may be mistakenly ruled out when reading and writing assessments are not sensitive enough to detect visual sensory impairments (e.g., right hemispatial neglect in clients with left hemisphere dysfunction).

WORKING MEMORY IN READING AND WRITING

A wide range of daily language-related activities have been linked to working memory ability in adults. These include writing, note-taking, following directions, reasoning, and learning (Engle et al., 1999; Gathercole, 1999). Therefore, working memory should be routinely assessed and treated in clients with both central and peripheral reading and writing disorders. One component of the ABRS involves repetition of nonwords. Nonword repetition is an indicator of phonological working memory (Baddeley et al., 1999; Gathercole, 1999) because it relies on the ability to store and retrieve an unfamiliar sequence of sounds. When recognition of letters and words is delayed clients rely heavily on working memory as they decode words in a LBL fashion. The speech-language pathologist is encouraged to examine auditory and visual working memory ability during testing and specific treatment activities. Does the client frequently forget what he or she has just heard, said, seen, read or written? Does the client need working memory training in order to make use of the LBL reading strategy, or to use the inner speech strategy? Can he or she write a word to dictation that he or she just copied? See pages 63, 65, and 69 for further discussion of how working memory can be addressed when treating peripheral reading and writing disorders. The remainder of this chapter is devoted to specific treatment methods and tools that address peripheral reading and writing disorders in the context of visual system dysfunction.

TREATMENT OF ACQUIRED PERIPHERAL READING AND WRITING DISORDERS

Clients with significant visual system dysfunction may have difficulty responding to formal language tests (e.g., the Boston Naming Test [Kaplan, Goodglass, & Weintraub, 2001], the RCBA-2 [LaPointe & Horner, 2006]). Visual acuity and auditory comprehension may be adequate and yet they are unable to follow instructions to look at, find, or point to pictures, objects, and words. Occasionally, a client may even report that he or she is unable to see, read, or write anything despite contradictory evidence, or complain that his or her glasses do not work anymore. In some cases, attempts at copying or writing reveal the inability to initiate writing movements, prolonged staring, or withdrawal behavior. Modification of the size, font, and format of picture or graphic material may be needed. When reflexive blinking is infrequent the reader should be encouraged to blink intermittently while reading. This refreshes the graphic image presented to the photoreceptors (Tse, Baumgarten, & Greenlee, 2010) and can improve letter and word recognition. One particularly astute client with bilateral parietal-occipital strokes described his method of reading short phrases by intermittently closing his eyes. This allowed him to begin again with better word recognition. He called this strategy the *relax method*: "I thought of using the relax method for two to three words (closes eyes), then quickly do it again (opens and closes eyes) so it becomes a sentence. This seems to slow it down and settle it down."

Adjusting the cognitive load and the balance between auditory and visual stimuli within language activities may also improve client responsiveness. For example, while the client is engaged in basic visual language tasks such as matching letters or words, reducing the amount of verbal instruction may improve visual attention to task. An errorless learning strategy is helpful at this point such as presenting a single letter, word, or picture, telling the client what it is and asking him her to locate it and then name the letter again.

Some readers move or bob their head as they try to locate objects or words; they may perform searching movements with their hands rather than their eyes, due to impaired visual motor of visual spatial skills. Sometimes this inefficient search strategy can be extinguished by instructing the client to reach out and grasp word cards or objects. If he or she repeatedly misses the target when reaching or searches with his or her hands instruct him or her to "make your eyes tell your hand what to do." In some cases, after several tries the head bobbing will be extinguished and the client will be able to direct his or her gaze and fixate objects and words more easily and accurately (author observation). When symptoms associated with Balint syndrome are noted (e.g., simultanagnosia, gaze apraxia, optic ataxia, difficulty fixating letters, words, or pictures), using a relatively smaller visual target is more likely to elicit a response (Devinsky & D'Esposito, 2004). Enclosing words in a border helps clients to see the stimulus as a whole rather than as separate bits of information (Myers, 1999). As previously noted, consultation with an occupational therapist is beneficial when these maladaptive search behaviors are observed.

Improving Visual Scanning for Reading

Occupational therapists often engage clients in activities that elicit broader saccadic eye movements. The goal is to survey the physical environment as a whole, and to understand the relationships between objects within the space (Zihl, 2000). Activities that elicit larger saccades in a left-to-right gaze shifting pattern may increase the range of eye movements for reading in clients with a visual field cut, hemispatial neglect, or ocular apraxia. Visual fields are measured in degrees. Imagine a band encircling the head at pupil level, with a total of 360 degrees in circumference. The normal visual field span is 150 degrees for each eye; that is 90 degrees from each pupil towards the ear, and 70 degrees from each pupil toward the nose. A minimum of two degrees on the left and right sides of the fixation point is necessary to cover text that spans 10 to 12 letters at a distance of 25 cm. For readers with hemianopia, a minimum of five degrees to the left and right of fixation is needed for normal reading (Gillen, 2009). Treatment of reading disorders in hemianopic clients should address visual attention skills; the frequency and size of saccadic movements into the hemianopic field, including small-scale eye movements for reading; and the organization of visual search and scan eye movements (Goodwin, 2014; Kerkhoff, 2000).

Simple matching tasks may be used to elicit a left-right scan pattern. For example, place a block-printed word card to the left of midline and several sentence cards to the right of midline (e.g. Descripto Cards [Communication Skill Builders]). The clinician instructs the client to match the single word card at the left with the sentence card that contains the target word to the right. When word cards are placed atop an open three-ring binder, the three rings act as both a tactile and visual midline landmark.

Another exercise to promote right-left-right reading saccades is the alphabet saccades activity, which pairs sound-letter integration with gaze shifts (i.e., saccades). The client scans lines of letters to locate a target letter or underlines each letter while saying the associated sound. The format of the 13 printable worksheets is tailored for younger subjects, but this type of activity is appropriate for adult readers with a reduced range of eye movements, hemianopia, or hemispatial neglect. These worksheets may be downloaded from the website (www.eyecanlearn.com) and used as a warmup task for other reading and writing exercises. The super saccades activity elicits saccadic eye movements also. In the number saccades exercise, clients name numbers as they appear in randomly spaced intervals.

The clinician may also use pen-and-paper, open-ended phrase- or sentence-completion tasks in multiple choice format such as those found in *Therapy Guide for Language and Speech Disorders, Volume 1* (Kilpatrick, 1977), or other exercises that elicit a left-to-right scan pattern such as *Lessons for the Right Brain: Reading, Writing & Visual Processing* (Baines & Miller, 2014). Verbal cues to "move your eyes toward the left (right or downward) to find the number (letter or word)" and intensive small-scale scanning practice in the context of reading exercises helps increase client awareness of items in the neglected or unattended space (author observation). For higher-level clients, combining visual scanning tasks with mental reasoning or memory exercises will increase the cognitive challenge. For example, in a paper-and-pencil task, the client reads and then adds a series of coin amounts (e.g. four pennies, three nickels, five dimes, three quarters; see Bressler-Richardson, 1996) while recalling sentences of increasing length and complexity (see Martinoff, Martinoff, & Stoke, 1981). After tallying the coins, the client repeats the target sentence. This activity may improve client awareness of hemispatial neglect or inattention, or reduce omission errors and difficulty scanning in the horizontal direction.

Improving Recognition of Letter and Word Forms

Lesions of the ventral or central visual pathway impair recognition of letters and words (alexia), static forms (agnosia), and faces (prosopagnosia) despite normal visual acuity (Fahle & Greenlee, 2003; Gillen, 2009). Agnosia for letters and words limits the reader's access to the orthographic lexicon, the long term memory for words accessed through semantic, phonological and visual orthographic input (Beeson, Rewega, Vail, & Rapcsak, 2000). The ability to recognize and name upper- and lowercase letters is a key component of reading and spelling. These skills are associated with phonemic awareness (Wood & McLemore, 2001) and are strong predictors of the ability to learn to read in first graders. Letter naming remains a strong predictor of reading ability in fourth-grade readers (Adams, 1990; Honig, 1996; Riley, 1996).

Neuropsychologist Josef Zihl (2000) reported on the treatment of letter recognition in two adult clients. Client One had sustained a closed head injury and had chronic hypoxia; Client Two had experienced bilateral occipitotemporal infarctions. Both had left homonymous hemianopia and agnosia resulting in the inability to recognize faces, objects or letters such that neither client was able to read. In Zihl's study, the subjects were trained to identify distinctive features of letters, objects and faces, and to develop "cognitive strategies to supervise and control visual identification" using an errorless learning strategy (Wilson & Evans, 1996). Following oculomotor scanning training to improve the range of eye movements, each subject intensively practiced discriminating visually distinct uppercase letter pairs (I vs O) for 980 to 1660 trials; letter pairs that had features in common (I vs T) for 1160 to 2140 trials; and very similar letters (E vs F) for 740 to 1540 trials. Client One showed significant improvement in recognition of letters with common features and letters that were very similar, while Client Two showed significant improvement in recognition of all three categories of letters. An unexpected finding was that as letter identification improved whole word recognition also improved.

We learn letter names and letter identities in a conventional order, the *alphabet line* (Berteletti, Lucangeli, & Zorzi, 2012). Hamilton and Sanford (1978) established that English speaking subjects run through sections of the alphabet line in a subvocalic manner when making decisions about letter order in the alphabet. Using the alphabet line as a tool for identification and association of letter shapes with letter names is useful for both decoding words and for spelling and writing words in cases of pure alexia (author observation). Clients who cannot recognize, match, or name letters should be given a set of upper- and lowercase alphabet cards for homework practice. When there is damage to the visual word form area, clients often trace the letters on paper, their palm, or in the air in order to identify them. Letter identification practice should continue as long as letter and word recognition are impaired. Eventually, it may be possible for some individuals to internalize this strategy and mentally trace or sequence the letters. A study by neuropsychologist G.M. Reicher (1969) found that letter discrimination is superior when letters are presented in word context. Based on this finding, a practice drill that requires the client to decide which of two visually similar words (e.g. HEAD and HEAT) contains a specific letter (T) may improve letter recognition in some clients.

Phonics Genius App

There are a number of apps that provide unlimited practice in letter and word recognition. The Phonics Genius app (AlligatorApps.com) allows for the creation of custom word categories. Individual words such as minimal pairs with final T or D may be entered in the Customize Flashcards component found in Settings. Click on Customize Flashcards, click the (+) sign, and then click Create New List. Name the category (e.g., Minimal Pairs) and then click Save. This new category will show up on the Home Screen at the end of the series of target phoneme selections. To add printed words to your new category, in Settings click on Customize Flashcards; find the new category you added at the bottom of the list of phoneme categories and click on it; click the (+) sign, and type the word you want to enter. Record yourself saying the word and click Save. Type the letter(s) you want highlighted and click Save. After all words are entered into the category you created, click Save again. In Settings select Play Mode and select Listening–Identify the correct word from a list of two words. The client is instructed to select which of two printed words matches the verbal model. Customizing this app for therapy and homework practice takes a bit of time but provides unlimited practice in the discrimination of visually similar words. Add words two at a time, so that letter and word identities may be mastered before moving on to new letters and minimal pairs. See pages 63 to 64 for further discussion of the Phonics Genius app. This app is available for iPad, iPad Touch, and iPhone but not Android devices.

Build-A-Word Express App

The Build-A-Word Express app (www.atreks.com) provides exercises in matching upper- or lowercase letters to letter names in order to spell up to 1290 words. Letters are selected from a random group of letters using a point-and-touch gesture. The client hears the name of each letter when he touches it. Correct letter choices immediately slide into a slot in the word; incorrect letter choices are audible, but remain static. One advantage to the Build-A-Word Express app is that word lists may be customized. Disadvantages are that there are no picture stimuli, there is no option to present the entire alphabet, and the app is available for iPhone and iPad, but not Android devices. The graphics and sounds are designed for ages 6 to 8 but in my experience, they are not off-putting for the adult client. Within-app purchases are available to expand word lists.

Using the Alphabet Line as a Spelling Strategy

The Tactus Therapy Writing app (Tactus Therapy Solutions, Ltd.) provides practice in the identification of upper- or lowercase letters and written spelling. In the Spell What You See and Spell What You Hear components, clients select and sequence letters in response to pictures or audible words. Word length varies from 3 to 10 letters and vocabulary lists can be personalized. There are three levels of difficulty to choose from (easy, medium, hard). In the hard setting, letter selections are made from the entire alphabet presented in two rows of letter tiles. Letter tiles are selected and placed one-by-one in a series of blank spaces to spell the target word. Each time the client touches the letter tile he or she hears the letter name. Responses may be checked before being entered, at which time incorrect letter choices are automatically removed prompting the client to begin again. There is a Copy mode for clients who cannot retrieve or maintain mental images of letters and words that provides errorless learning practice. The Tactus Therapy Writing app trains sound-letter association and alphabetic sequence, and it promotes scanning into the left and right visual fields as the reader searches for letters. Random searching for letters is avoided by instructing the client to "dive in" and touch any letter he or she sees, and then proceed through the alphabet until he or she locates the target letter by name (i.e., auditory cue) if not by sight. Letter targets are gradually associated with a "neighborhood" of letters within the alphabet line and retrieved more quickly (author observation). Tactus Language Therapy apps are available for both Apple and Android devices.

LINGRAPHICA TALKPATH APPS

Lingraphica TalkPath: Writing

The Lingraphica TalkPath app (www.aphasia.com) Writing component has both Copying and Spelling elements. In the Spelling element, Level One, the client is prompted to "Spell the pictured word" after hearing a word associated with the picture (e.g., "meal" with picture of food). All words have four letters. The client then locates highlighted uppercase letters in either a QWERTY keyboard or in the alphabet line to spell the target word. At Level Two, letters are not highlighted, and the client chooses them from the entire alphabet. Blank spaces indicate the number of letters in the word. Levels Three and Four present six-letter, and seven- or eight-letter words, respectively and contain more irregularly spelled words. This app is only available for the iPad.

The Phonics Genius, Build-a-Word Express, Tactus Therapy-Writing, and Lingraphica TalkPath-Writing apps are excellent tools for the treatment of letter recognition, letter matching, letter naming, and written spelling in acquired alexia. When these peripheral reading skills become more automatic through intensive practice, cognitive resources are freed up for use in other components of reading such as working memory for sounds in words (Lott, Carney, Glezer, & Friedman, 2010), and reading comprehension.

Lingraphica TalkPath: Memory-Number Recall

Clients with left neglect or those with simultanagnosia may benefit from practice with the Lingraphica TalkPath Immediate Memory-Number Recall component. At Level Two, stimuli consist of 1 1/4 inch high, two-digit numbers. The client is tasked with viewing and remembering the two-digit number and then stating or typing the number following a brief delay. Clients with left neglect or stimultanagnosia may reply "2" in response to the graphic number 42. The clinician then covers the number two and asks the client to try again. Just as the client recognizes the number four, the clinician uncovers the number two. In this manner, some clients with simultanagnosia can briefly recognize the two-digit number (author observation). This exercise may be replicated with word stimuli and is easily adapted to print when an iPad is not available. Educating the client about the nature of his or her visual sensory impairment (e.g., that numbers, letters, words, or objects may appear and then disappear from conscious awareness) and providing intensive practice may improve visual recognition of numbers and letters in clients with simultanagnosia.

MakeChange App

The MakeChange app (slidetorock.com) repeatedly prompts the client to locate pennies, nickels, dimes, and quarters by scanning left to right across the top of the iPad screen. He or she selects coins equal to a given amount and draws them down to the bottom of the screen. Clients with left neglect or simultanagnosia may be aware of a coin at one instance, and then be unable to find it the next moment. Repeatedly locating coins, placing them at the bottom of the screen, and then scanning left to right to find and count them again may improve recognition and discrimination of coins and increase the range and efficiency of visual scanning for near functional language activities.

Gaze is forcibly tied to the target of a pointing movement and is anchored to that point of focus until the arm movement changes (Neggers & Bekkering, 2001). The paired eye and hand movements associated with these apps (e.g., scanning followed by touch to select and place letter, tiles, or coins) may help to reestablish the gaze-shift + fixation pattern of reading saccades, increase attention to word boundaries, and improve visual search in the context of reading and other functional activities. In cases of object- and stimulus-centered neglect, where parts of words are omitted in both the left and right visual fields, these exercises draw the reader's attention to the beginning and ending of words (see Table 2-1). These apps are useful components of a client's home exercise program or may be used as warmup exercises in language therapy sessions.

Improving Attention to Sound and Letter Sequences

Phonological Awareness and Working Memory

Phonological awareness is an important correlate of learning to read (Beeson et al, 2010; Dehaene, 2011). Treatment that focuses on working memory for a sequence of letter names, phonemes, or syllables strengthens working memory for sequences of graphemes in oral and written spelling. English speakers use inner speech to rehearse or review sequences of letter names as words are deciphered (Hamilton & Sanford, 1978). Memory decay is avoided through subvocalization or silent rehearsal of letter names or sequences of items that form a memory trace in the phonological buffer (Baddeley, 2000). When word recognition is delayed due to poor letter recognition the reader with pure alexia must rely on auditory memory for sound-letter correspondences during the slow decoding of words.

Several apps are available to retrain phonological awareness and auditory-verbal memory. The Auditory Processing Studio app (Virtual Speech Center, Inc.) has three components:

- *Auditory Discrimination* trains clients to identify sounds in initial, medial, and final word positions and to discriminate minimal pairs (bit-fit-sit).
- *Phonological Awareness* trains clients to identify the number of phonemes and syllables in words and blend them to make single syllable and multisyllabic words.
- *Auditory Closure* focuses on the generation of missing elements of words and sentences.

Each of these tasks engages the phonological working memory component of language.

The Phonics Genius app (AlligatorApps.com) (See page 61) is designed to develop phonological awareness in early readers by training them to hear the individual sounds in words. It also may be used to train immediate auditory recall. The app groups words into 225 categories based on initial, medial, and final sounds. The 6000 word stimuli range from 3 to 13 letters. There are four different font styles in upper- or lowercase letters. The color of the target letters in each word may be changed in Settings to provide contrast with the rest of the word. In Play Mode-Game, the reader is presented with an array of two to six words; the target letters are in a contrasting color. The reader selects the word that matches the auditory model. The Phonics Genius app is appropriate for the adult client with acquired peripheral dyslexia who cannot discriminate visually similar words or who fails to detect the initial, medial, or final letters within words due to hemianopia, allocentric neglect, impaired recognition of letter and word forms, poor phonological awareness, or impaired memory for the sequence of sounds in words.

In cases of pure alexia and multimodal alexia, the Phonics Genius app provides endless practice in identifying and discriminating letters and bigrams (i.e., common letter pairs) and words, within and across phonetic categories. The app may be set to loop across all phonetic categories so that word length and the location of target sounds and letters within words varies unpredictably (e.g., me*ch*anic, *ch*amomile, stoma*ch*), prompting the alexic or hemianopic client to carefully scan word boundaries. Personalized word lists may be created by adding a new category of words and recording a verbal model of each word. This app is easily adapted to a modified Copy and Recall Treatment (CART) protocol (Beeson et al., 2002) where clients are instructed to read the word, spell it aloud several times, copy it three times, and then write it from memory. Any of these apps that present both regularly and irregularly spelled words of increasing length are appropriate for clients with a phonological buffer or orthographic buffer (i.e., visuospatial sketchpad) deficit, and for those clients who exhibit a word length effect (i.e., increase in errors with longer words).

INCORPORATING MOVEMENT INTO LANGUAGE REHABILITATION

Letter-by-Letter Reading and the Tactile Kinesthetic Strategy

The inability to name letters limits the alexic client's ability to use the LBL reading strategy (Mozzo & Caramazza, 1998). The reader must rely on a tactile or kinesthetic strategy for recognizing letters (e.g., air tracing with head or finger). This tracing behavior was first documented by Goldstein and Gelb (1918) in a World War I veteran who had sustained lesions to the posterior skull and to the left parietal-occipital junction, and later in a client with mercury poisoning (Landis et al., 1982). James and Gauthier (2006) examined the relationship between visual perception of letters and cortical areas associated with letter writing. They found that tracing letters recruited areas of the cortex associated with the visual perception of letters. The converse was also true, that is, letter perception recruited the part of the motor cortex associated with writing letters. Lott et al. (2010) demonstrated that some clients with fluent aphasia and phonological alexia benefit from intensive practice using a tactile-kinesthetic strategy (i.e., tracing letters into client's palm) to identify letters. The authors concluded that this reinforcement of the LBL reading strategy may be used to decode both trained and untrained words and can lead to the ability to read sentences in some individuals.

Paired Eye and Hand Movements in Reading

A treatment strategy that pairs arm and hand movements with reading is supported by several studies that examined eye movements during pointing and reaching tasks. One study of 18 healthy adults found that gaze is forcibly tied to the target of a pointing movement and is anchored to that point of focus until the arm movement changes (Neggers & Bekkering, 2001). The authors theorized that this pairing of eye and arm movements was coordinated at the level of the superior colliculi in the brainstem. In a review of studies related to eye movement in everyday activities, Land (2006) concluded that hand movements are led by eye movements: "It has been pointed out repeatedly that each type of action has its own associated regime of eye movements, and that fixations on objects tend to precede actions upon them by up to a second."

In my experience, incorporating a hand movement into reading tasks can increase the range of eye movements into the affected field for reading in some clients with impaired reading saccades. This may be accomplished by instructing clients to point to, circle, or underline each word as they read when doing paper-and-pencil tasks. When combined with verbal cues to "use your eyes to guide your hand movements," "keep your eyes moving," or to "point your eyes at each word" performance on simple matching, scanning and reading activities improves in some clients (author observation). The Lingraphica TalkPath app Writing component (http://www.aphasia.com) and the Tactus Writing app Fill-in-the-Blank, Copy, Spell What You Hear, and Spell What You See components (Tactus Therapy Solutions, Ltd.) pair a gesture (e.g., manual letter selection and letter tile placement) with searching for letters across the alphabet line. The left-right-left scan pattern may become more regular and efficient through clinician instruction and practice.

The Visuospatial Sketchpad and Orthographic Memory

The visuospatial sketchpad (i.e., graphemic or orthographic buffer) serves working memory for writing and typing. Recent functional Magnetic Resonance Imaging findings suggest that the primary visual cortex (V1) is the site of the visuospatial sketchpad because it responds to both verbal and episodic memory tasks in an amodal fashion (Likova, 2014). Words are retrieved from long-term memory and held briefly in the visuospatial sketchpad until they are converted to letter names (in oral spelling) and to graphemes (in written spelling) (Menichelli et al., 2012; Purcell, Napoliello, & Eden, 2011). Baddeley (2003) suggests that the role of the visuospatial sketchpad in reading is to support visual imagery of the printed page and help the reader easily scan from one line of print to the next. It may also help the reader retain a visual image of letter sequences during LBL reading and written spelling (Beeson, 2004). Writing or typing to dictation with words and sentences of increasing length engages both phonological working memory and orthographic memory.

INTERACTIVE TREATMENT PROTOCOLS

Anagram and Copy Treatment & Copy and Recall Treatment

Interactive treatment protocols promote interaction between phonological and lexical (orthographic) spelling routes (Aftonomos, Steele, & Wertz, 1997; Beeson, 2004; Beeson & Egnor, 2006; Beeson, Rising, Kim, & Rapcsak, 2010). Treatment that engages both phonological and orthographic spelling systems has been shown to reduce semantic spelling errors in a client with a left frontal stroke (Hillis, Rapp, & Caramazza, 1999). Two examples of interactive language therapy protocols are Anagram and Copy Treatment (ACT) and CART (Beeson et al., 2002; http://www.aphasia.arizona.edu). ACT is intended to strengthen the mental image of written words by sequencing letter tiles to spell target words and copying them to reinforce their spelling. CART protocol pairs picture and word stimuli. Clients identify pictured objects, spell the object name aloud, copy target words multiple times, and then write them from memory. Each set of five target words is mastered before moving on to the next set. These two treatment methods are described in an article by Beeson (2004), published in *Topics in Stroke Rehabilitation*. Positive treatment effects in aphasia have been demonstrated for both protocols (Beeson, Hirsch, & Rewega, 2002). Multiple copying trials and then writing target words from memory may also reinforce the process of converting phonemes to allographs and the associated motor programs for writing (Beeson & Rapcsak, 2002) in clients with acquired dysgraphia.

Recently ACT and CART treatment protocols were combined with the Tactus Writing Therapy app procedure. In an interactive treatment study, Beeson, Higginson, & Rising (2013) compared the response to CART vs T-CART (texting on a QWERTY keyboard) in a client with aphasia and apraxia. Training alternated between CART and T-CART with three sets of five words for each training method. Although learning was demonstrated for each treatment method the client retained more words with the CART protocol. The authors suggest that further research is needed with combined CART and T-CART training.

Some of these therapy activities were developed for the treatment of aphasia but may be adapted to the treatment of peripheral reading and writing disorders such as pure alexia, hemianopic alexia, or peripheral agraphias. Treatment goals would include improving letter recognition, strengthening mental representations of single words, and improving graphomotor function for individual letters and words by copying and writing words from memory. Further studies of the efficacy of ACT, CART, and other interactive treatments for both central and peripheral acquired reading disorders are needed.

TRANSITIONING TO TEXT-BASED READING IN ALEXIA

When deciding on a treatment plan, it is important to introduce word matching, phrase- and sentence-completion, and word reordering tasks even as clients are still learning to recognize letters. This provides a lexical and semantic context that may facilitate recognition of familiar letter sequences, whole words, and word sequences. However, even very basic reading tasks such as multiple-choice phrase completion may place excessive visual and cognitive demands on the client with a peripheral reading disorder. This is particularly true when both visual sensory and visual motor systems are involved (e.g. visual field loss, agnosia for letters and words, impaired reading saccades).

Lingraphica TalkPath App

The Lingraphica TalkPath app Writing component, scrambled sentences exercise, guides the client toward text-level reading. The client is instructed to sequence three or more words in order to form a sentence. As he or she touches and selects each word, he or she hears the verbal form of the word. The client may elect to hear the entire sentence read aloud in order to make adjustments in word order. Stimuli are presented across five levels of difficulty with words and sentences of increasing length and complexity. The Complete the Phrase component combines a letter decoding task with a sentence-completion and written spelling task for the pure alexic client who uses LBL reading. This activity also can lead to improvement in auditory memory and help the client with impaired word recognition match the auditory trace of a word with its graphic form.

Sentence unscrambling activities provide clues to word order (e.g., number of words in sentence, first word is capitalized, punctuation indicates last word in sentence) and reveal a client's residual knowledge of orthography, syntax and punctuation. For example, a 64-year-old client with global alexia following left temporal-parietal-occipital hemorrhagic stroke reported: "I know that's [the word] 'I' because it's only one [meaning the letter stands alone]"; "That word goes at the beginning because it's a big [capital] letter"; and "The period means that this word goes at the end." While there is limited evidence of carryover of single word training to reading phrases, sentences or paragraphs (Cherney, 2004; Kim & Lemke, 2016; Lacey et al, 2010) treatment should capitalize on these types of clues to engage top-down language processes that will help the client with pure alexia transition to text-level reading.

Multiple Oral Reading Method and Oral Reading for Language in Aphasia

Two treatment methods that target text-level reading in acquired alexia are the Multiple Oral Reading (MOR) method (Beeson, 1998; Beeson & Insalaco, 1998; Moyer, 1979); and Oral Reading for Language in Aphasia (ORLA) (Cherney, Merbitz, & Grip, 1986). MOR is intended to reduce reliance on the LBL reading strategy (Moyer, 1979) with multiple readings of the same connected paragraphs supported by clinician cues to word identity and pronunciation. It is hypothesized that the semantic and syntactic content of text-level reading improves the reader's access to the orthographic lexicon, thereby enhancing whole word recognition (Beeson & Insalaco, 1998).

Clinician and client perform choral reading of passages when using the ORLA protocol. The client eventually transitions to independent oral reading. Positive outcomes in reading rate and oral reading accuracy following ORLA and MOR treatments have been demonstrated across studies and alexia types (e.g., mixed, pure, phonological, and deep alexia) (Cherney, 2004; Kim & Russo, 2010; Lacey et al, 2007; Mayer & Murray, 2002). However, reports of improvement in reading comprehension at the text level are limited. Joyce West, a professor of speech, language, and hearing sciences at Lehman College in New York, presented a single case study poster session on alexia without agraphia (ASHA, 2009; Session 1823, Poster 202). West's client had sustained a left parietal lobe contusion and used the LBL reading strategy. West described a modified MOR protocol that resulted in a significant improvement in reading rate, the client's ability to recognize his own writing and to read and comprehend newspapers and novels. The striking improvement in text-level reading in this case may be due to the milder nature of the injury relative to clients with more significant cortical lesions.

ORLA may also improve visual scanning for reading. Kim, Rising, Rapcsak, & Beeson (2015) used eye tracking measures to study the effect of 12 weeks of combined MOR and ORLA treatment in a 42-year-old male client with chronic anomic aphasia and central alexia nine years post left hemisphere stroke. The client also worked with a comparable oral-reading home program for 23 hours. Eye tracking measures were taken pre- and post-treatment. In normal reading, fixations tend to be located just to the left of the middle of a word regardless of word length (Rayner, 1979; Spitzyna et al., 2007). Prior to treatment, the client in this study first fixated closer to the beginning of the word. Post-treatment first fixation position moved toward the middle of the word. Other improvements included an increase in oral reading accuracy and reading rate for overlearned passages as well as increased reading rate for new passages. Consistent with other studies of MOR, reading comprehension did not improve. Further studies are needed to determine which alexic clients will benefit most from MOR, ORLA, or combined treatments for LBL reading in cases of acquired alexia and agraphia. Beeson, Magloire, and Robey (2005) suggest that some clients need strong letter processing skills in order to show positive outcomes following MOR treatment.

Optokinetic Stimulation and Text-Level Reading in Hemianopic Alexia

Clients with unilateral and bilateral hemianopia report slow visual processing and typically have eye movements that are inadequate to compensate for their visual field loss (i.e., hypometric saccades) in the ipsilateral, contralateral, or in both directions, which leads to hemianopic alexia. Optokinetic stimulation (OKS), a graphic display moving toward the left elicits a quick saccade toward the right hemianopic field without conscious awareness. OKS has been used as a bottom-up approach to retraining eye movements in hemianopic dyslexia (Leff & Starrfelt, 2014) and in the treatment of visual spatial attention in neglect dyslexia (Pizzamiglio et al, 1998). When the eyes follow a moving object in a leftward direction (i.e., smooth pursuit movement) the optokinetic reflex triggers a quick saccade in the opposite direction allowing the viewer to keep the head stable

(Roeser, Valent, & Hosford-Dunn, 2007). OKS has led to changes in several types of neglect including body midline perception, distortion in line bisection, size estimation, and auditory neglect (Kerkhoff & Schenk, 2012). Treatment protocols are not consistent across studies of OKS making it difficult to draw conclusions about treatment efficacy (Kerkhoff et al, 2006; Pizzamiglio et al, 1990; Reinhart, Schindler, & Kerkhoff, 2011).

Readers with hemianopia begin to process semantic content before viewing the entire word. This leads them to guess at word identity and impairs reading comprehension. A number of studies of OKS using so-called Times Square leftward scrolling text have shown positive treatment outcomes in hemianopic dyslexia including an increase in the range of eye movements into the affected field, improved reading saccades, shorter fixation times, fewer reading errors, and an increase in reading speed (Spitzyna et al., 2007). Josef Zihl (1995a, 2000) trained left hemianopic clients to attend to the beginning of every word and trained right hemianopic clients to attend to the end of every word when viewing leftward scrolling text. Positive outcomes included fewer prefix and suffix omission errors. Measures of reading comprehension are generally not reported in these studies. Methods for incorporating OKS into the treatment of acquired dyslexia and further studies of the best method for delivering OKS are needed. A sample passage presented in Times Square scrolling text can be found at http://www.eyecanlearn.com.

The "Read-Right" program uses moving text that scrolls from right to left to trigger the optokinetic reflex. Woodhead et al. (2015) used this web-based research and training platform to study whether persons with homonymous hemianopia and hemianopic alexia would demonstrate improved reading speed after treatment via the Read-Right treatment program. The authors were able to demonstrate that the Read-Right program, "improves text reading speed in hemianopic patients, but not in participants matched for slow text reading but without hemianopia." These studies illustrate the need for more evidence-based research as well as individualized treatment programs for acquired, peripheral reading disorders. The reader may learn more about the Read-Right program at: http://www.readright.ucl.ac.uk/help/h_vft.php

Closed Captioning in Acquired Alexia Treatment

Closed captions are subtitles presented in the same language as television or movie audio/visual content. Closed captioning was first studied in the deaf and hearing-impaired populations (Markham, 1999). Researchers found significant benefits to general comprehension of video material when combined with captioning for these populations (Jensema, 1996; Schmidt & Haydu, 1992; Withrow, 1994). Similar results were found in a random sample of hearing-impaired older adults when closed captioning was combined with hearing aid use (Gordon-Salant & Callahan, 2010).

Close captioning of video material has also been shown to improve reading comprehension in normal hearing, native English speakers, with notable improvements in vocabulary, word recognition, and overall reading comprehension skills (Goldman & Goldman, 1988; Griffin & Dumestre, 1993; Koskinen, Wilson, & Jensema 1985; Wilson & Jensema, 1985). Watching captioned television programs has also been shown to improve the ability to process running text in both verbal and written modalities in persons learning English as a second language (ESL) (Vanderplank, 1988).

Clients with visual system dysfunction often report that they are no longer interested in watching television, or that they "can't keep up" or follow a storyline following a stroke (author observation). In normal aging, hearing loss, visual motor, and visual sensory impairments may compound the decline in ability to ignore irrelevant information (Kemper & McDowd, 2006) and to quickly process scene changes.

With these thoughts in mind, it is important to consider closed captioning as a rehabilitation strategy for persons with acquired alexia. There is likely to be a minimal level of auditory and literacy competency for readers to benefit from closed captioning (Danan, 2004), as well as for the ability to shift attention between auditory, visual, and text input. Captioning speed is typically

141 words/minute (Gordon-Salant & Callahan, 2010), and may be too rapid for some persons with acquired alexia to process the captioned text. Nevertheless, closed captioning benefits some individuals, and merits further exploration as a treatment strategy for acquired peripheral and central reading disorders.

TREATMENT OF ACQUIRED PERIPHERAL AGRAPHIAS

An important goal of the writing assessment is to distinguish between the peripheral and central components of writing (Grainger & Holcomb, 2009; Purcell, Turkeltaub, et al., 2011). See Table 2-3 for error patterns associated with central and peripheral dysgraphias. When a client presents with both peripheral and central writing disorders, the peripheral writing impairment must be addressed first in order to achieve maximum benefit from treatment of the central language deficit (Beeson & Rapcsak, 2002). Clients with central agraphias have difficulty writing words and sentences due to damage to the phonological and/or semantic routes for written spelling, leaving them unable to retrieve graphic word forms from the orthographic lexicon. Peripheral dysgraphias are attributed to multiple causes including:

- Loss of access to specific motor sequences associated with letter formation (i.e., the size and order of the writing movements)
- Visuospatial impairment (e.g., coordinating egocentric and allocentric frames of reference, coordinating eye-hand movements)
- Visual motor impairments (e.g., disruption of saccades, dysconjugate gaze)
- Visual sensory deficits (e.g., visual field loss, impaired contrast sensitivity, impaired form or color vision)
- Constructional deficits

Treatment should be individualized for each client to address the specific barriers to written communication. Referral to occupational therapy is crucial when signs or symptoms of visual system dysfunction are noted. Graphomotor function is also typically assessed and treated by occupational therapy.

Apps such as Tracing Letters, Cursive Writing, and Cursive Words (Horizon Business, Inc.) provide structured practice in printing and writing script in lower- and uppercase with either hand. They may be used as a warmup for writing tasks in speech therapy, or as a component of a home exercise program. Treatment might alternate between the Cursive Writing app and a whiteboard app such as Doodle Buddy (Dinopilot) for practice writing target words from memory or for spontaneous writing. The Doodle Buddy app has the option of emailing writing samples or messages to the clinician or family and friends. Appendix D provides a lesson plan for retraining typing skills for clients for whom typing (hunt and peck or bimanual) is a more functional method of written communication. The overall treatment goal is to establish motor plans for writing or typing so that more cognitive resources are available for retrieval of written spelling and for sentence formulation.

Using Augmentative Communication Apps to Treat Acquired Dysgraphia

When the motor act of writing is too challenging, or when written expression is limited due to a combination of central and peripheral writing impairments, augmentative and alternative communication (AAC) apps serve as both remedial and compensatory treatment tools. The Assistive Express app (Kiat Ng, available on iTunes) is an easy-to-use text-to-speech app. Words are typed on a QWERTY keyboard or selected via the word prediction option. The app has adaptive learning such that new and often used vocabulary are added to the word prediction list. Favorite or commonly used sentences can also be stored for later use. The Assistive Express app helps the client with pure alexia or agraphia transition from writing or typing single words to sentence formulation. Treatment may begin with a writing-to-dictation task to engage phonological working memory, visual word discrimination (i.e., using the word prediction component) and visual scanning across the keyboard, and later transition to composing an email that can be sent from within the app. As part of a home exercise program, clients may compose phrases or sentences using the Assistive Express app and email them to the clinician or friends and family members (See also T-CART, pg. 65).

SUMMARY

In summary acquired reading disorders are heterogenous. Reading fluency relies on intact visual sensory (e.g., acuity, contrast sensitivity, form recognition) and visual motor skills (e.g., convergence, fixation, saccadic shifts); fundamental sublexical skills (e.g., knowledge of sound-letter and letter-sound correspondences); and higher-level cognitive skills (e.g., attention, working memory). The rehabilitation of reading and writing in the adult neurological client requires a broad assessment with an eye toward error patterns that differentiate central from peripheral acquired reading and writing disorders. Vision-related error patterns reflect the viewer's spatial reference frame (allocentric or egocentric), the visual pathway that is affected (ventral or dorsal), and the cognitive components involved (bottom-up or top-down processing). Deficits in bottom-up processing of form and line elements will have a negative impact on top-down visual language processes (Flowers et al 2004; Wolf, 2007). Comprehension of written language may be further compromised by attention deficits and phonological working memory impairment (Mayer & Murray, 2002). Consultation with occupational therapy and neuro-optometry is imperative when working with clients who exhibit signs or symptoms of visual system dysfunction.

Phonological awareness training improves working memory for sounds in words. This in turn benefits oral and written spelling, as well as the use of inner speech, a compensatory strategy for working memory in spelling and writing. Some treatment methods developed for central language impairments (e.g., aphasia) such as CART are easily adapted to the client with peripheral dyslexia and agraphia. Targeting treatment at the single word, phrase, and short sentence levels concurrently provides a richer context for reading remediation and engages top-down language processes, including knowledge of orthography, syntax, and punctuation. Finally, MOR training and AAC applications may provide a bridge from reading and writing single words to phrase- and sentence-length written expression for clients with acquired, peripheral reading and writing disorders.

GENERAL TREATMENT GUIDELINES

The following is a summary of treatment strategies for adult neurological clients with visual system dysfunction and associated peripheral reading and writing disorders. The reader is referred to Appendix C for a list of applications and online exercises for the treatment of acquired reading and writing disorders.

1. Refer all neurological clients for visual motor and visual sensory testing (Teasell, Salter, Cotoi, Brar, & Donais, 2013; VA DoD, 2010). This is accomplished through referral to an occupational therapist or behavioral neurooptometrist. Consultation with an occupational therapist or neurooptometrist for the evaluation and treatment of oculomotor impairments may improve reading outcomes (see Zihl, 2000, p. 137).

2. When referring clients to a behavioral neurooptometrist, request a functional visual examination. This includes testing of visual fields, binocular function, depth perception, and visual

spatial perception. Additional measures with strong relevance to reading include near-point-of-convergence, contrast sensitivity, and UFOV, (or visual span for reading).

3. Use the client's own reading glasses during testing. When they are not available, have over-the-counter glasses available in a variety of strengths.

4. Place test and treatment materials at an angle on an easel or atop a three-ring binder to avoid glare from overhead lights.

5. Incorporate visual rest into cognitive-communicative testing and treatment sessions.

6. Encourage blinking when clients stare without responding.

7. Enclose objects or words in a border. This helps clients to see the stimulus as a whole rather than as separate bits of information (Myers, 1999).

8. Cut a window in a three-by-five card to assist clients in reading a few words at a time, when more than one line of print is distracting to the client (Powell & Torgerson, 2011).

9. Listen carefully to client descriptions of their experience with reading and writing. Their comments often provide clues to which intervention strategy to use.

10. Attempt to extinguish head bobbing or searching head movements by pairing eye and hand movements. Instruct clients to use their eyes to guide their hand movements while reaching for word cards or objects. Warm up with basic repetitive tasks such as sorting a deck of cards into piles by color (black/red), then by suit (e.g., hearts, clubs). Consult with an occupational therapist regarding how to extinguish head bobbing.

11. When clients report that they are not able to read despite evidence to the contrary, cover one eye at a time during the reading assessment to determine whether they recognize letters and words better with one eye alone. Consult with occupational therapy regarding the use of occlusive patching.

12. For lower functioning clients who are unable to locate and recognize words and letters, present just one word at a time. When clients report that they are not able to read word cards, instruct them to "Name any letter you see." If they still cannot identify the word, tell them what the word is and then ask them to try to see it and read it aloud. In other words, use *errorless learning.*

13. Evaluate the client's ability to name and write letters to dictation, recite and then write the alphabetic sequence, and associate letters with phonemes and phonemes with letters.

14. Reading should be tested at the single word and sentence-length levels, and with article-length material in both single- and two-column (e.g., newspaper) formats, to rule out hemispatial neglect for reading in clients with either left or right hemisphere lesions.

15. Compare performance when reading paragraph-level text (e.g., RCBA-2 paragraph-picture matching subtest) vs functional reading tasks where key information needs to be searched out across a variety of formats (e.g, prescription, calendar, recipe) as in the RCBA-2 functional reading subtest (LaPointe & Horner, 2006).

16. Before beginning treatment of neglect dyslexia determine which type of neglect the patient has based on his or her error pattern (e.g., viewer-, object-, or stimulus-centered) (Appendix B).

17. When a client has difficulty recognizing or locating letters and words, use exercises that naturally incorporate numbers, letters, or words in a prescribed sequence (e.g., calendars, working with the alphabet line, alphabetized lists, crossword puzzles).

18. In cases of hemispatial neglect, encourage gaze shifts into the affected field by instructing clients to "point your eyes toward the left/right" rather than telling them to turn their head. Eye movements lead head movements in naturally occurring gaze shifting (Land, 2006).

19. Orient the client to the left and right visual fields by presenting word stimuli in an open, three-ring binder. The rings act as a visual and tactile cue to midline. Instruct the client to match word stimuli to the left to word and sentence stimuli at the right of the three rings.

20. When you suspect that a client's small-scale reading eye movements may be impaired, incorporate tracing, pointing, circling, or underlining movements within language activities. Combining eye and hand movements may facilitate eye movements into the affected field (Margolis, 2011). Circling and underlining marks give an indication of what was read and what was not. Consult with occupational therapy on methods to increase the range of eye movements into the affected field.

21. Clients with a letter naming deficit may benefit from instruction in a tactile-kinesthetic strategy for decoding words such as tracing, copying, and sequencing letters. Using an errorless, learning strategy, alternate between letter naming practice and tasks that involve sequencing, tracing, copying, and writing words of three to five letters.

22. Introduce word matching, phrase- and sentence-completion, and word reordering tasks even as clients are still learning to recognize letters.

23. Continue training the peripheral components of reading and writing (e.g., letter naming, reading eye movements, copying and writing letters) beyond the point of mastery, with the goal of increasing speed of word decoding.

24. Introduce exercises that increase attention to the beginning and ending of words (e.g., Sort and Copy exercises where words are sorted into one of two semantic categories and then copied), Build-A-Word Express app (www.atreks.com), or Phonics Genius app (www.alligatorapps.com), or present visually similar printed word pairs (e.g., water, waited) and instruct the client to point to the word you say.

25. Cursive Writing, Cursive Words, and Tracing Letters apps provide lower- and uppercase letters to trace. Use them as a warmup task for writing tasks, or to train motor plans for printing and writing.

26. When a client cannot write letters or spell written words, try using a keyboard. Sometimes typed spelling is superior to written or oral spelling.

27. When a client presents with both a peripheral and a central writing disorder the peripheral writing impairment must be addressed first in order to achieve maximum benefit from treatment of the central language deficit (Beeson & Rapcsak, 2002).

28. Introduce exercises to improve working memory for sounds in words (i.e., phonological buffer) so that silent rehearsal or inner speech may be used to refresh phonological memory when the reader uses the LBL reading or tactile-kinesthetic method to slowly decode words and phrases.

29. Interactive treatment methods such as ACT and CART (Beeson et al, 2002) can be used to establish a core written vocabulary set. CART may also reinforce motor plans for writing in peripheral dysgraphia (Beeson & Rapcsak, 2002). When a client uses the LBL reading method, but has great difficulty naming letters, eliminate the verbal component of CART (i.e. oral spelling/letter naming) to increase attention to the visual word forms. Extinguish spontaneous oral spelling if it leads to perseveration or confusion, but keep the copying and writing from memory components.

30. Transition from LBL reading to text-level reading using the MOR protocol; or augmentative and assistive therapy apps.

31. Closed captioning with television programs and movies may facilitate recognition of written words and assist in transitioning from single-word reading to text-level reading in higher-functioning readers with acquired dyslexia.

32. OKS is a potential therapy tool for transitioning to text-level reading in acquired dyslexia. When using OKS, it is important to draw client attention to the beginning of each word in cases of left hemianopia, and to the end of each word in cases of right hemianopia. There is a need for the development of scrolling text applications and programs at this time.

33. AAC apps can serve as both remedial and compensatory treatment tools in acquired alexia (e.g., pure alexia, global alexia) and dysgraphia. Simple AAC apps such as the Assistive Express app (Kiat Ng, available on iTunes) that have a word prediction component provide practice in recognition of single words and written or typed spelling. Favorite or often used phrases can be stored for future use, or emailed to the therapist, family, or friends.

REFERENCES

Adams, M. J. (1990). *Beginning to read: Thinking and learning about print.* Cambridge, MA: MIT Press.

Aftonomos, L. B., Steele, R. D., & Wertz, R. T. (1997). Promoting recovery in chronic aphasia with an interactive technology. *Archives of Physical Medicine and Rehabilitation, 78,* 841-846.

Baddeley, A. D. (2000). The episodic buffer: A new component of working memory? *Trends in Cognitive Science, 4*(11), 417-423.

Baddeley, A. D. (2003). Working memory and language: An overview. *Journal of Communication Disorders, 36,* 189-208.

Baddeley, A. D., Gathercole, S. E., & Papagno, C. (1998). The phonological loop as a language learning device. *Psychological Review, 105,* 158-173.

Baines, K., Martin, A., & McMartin Heeringa, H. (1999). *Assessment of language-related functional activities.* Austin, TX: Pro-ed.

Baines, K., & Miller, P. (2014). *Lessons for the right brain* (2nd ed.). Austin, TX: Pro-ed.

Bates, S., Kay, J., Code, C., Haslam, C., & Hollowell, B. (2010). 18 years on: What next for the PALPA. International *Journal of Speech-Language Pathology, 12*(3), 190-202.

Beeson, P. M. (1998). Treatment for letter-by-letter reading: A case study. In: N Helm-Estabrooks and A.L. Holland (Eds.). *Approaches to the Treatment of Aphasia* (pp. 153-177). San Diego, CA: Singular Publishing.

Beeson, P. M. (2004). Remediation of written language. *Topics in Stroke Rehabilitation, 11*(1), 37-48.

Beeson, P. M. and Egnor, H. (2006). Combining treatment for written and spoken naming. *Journal of International Neuropsychological Society, 12*(6), 816-827.

Beeson, P.M. & Insalaco, D. (1998). Acquired alexia: Lessons from successful treatment. *Journal of International Neuropsychological Society, 4,* 621-635.

Beeson, P. M., Rewega, M. A., Vail, S., & Rapcsak, S. Z. (2000). Problem solving approach to agraphia treatment: Interactive use of lexical and sublexical spelling routes. *Aphasiology, 14*(5/6), 551-565.

Beeson, P. M., & Rising, K. (2010). The Arizona Battery for Reading and Spelling. Retrieved from www.aphasia.arizona.edu/Aphasia_Research_Project/Assessment_Materials.html

Beeson, P. M., Higginson, K., & Rising, K. (2013). Writing treatment for aphasia: A texting approach. *Journal of Speech, Language, and Hearing Research, 56,* 945-955.

Beeson, P. M., Hirsch, F. M., & Rewega, M. A. (2002). Successful single word writing treatment: Experimental analyses of four cases. *Aphasiology, 14*(4-6), 473-491.

Beeson, P. M., Magloire, J. G., & Robey, R. (2005). Letter-by-letter reading: Natural recovery and response to treatment. *Behavioural Neurology, 16,* 191-192

Beeson, P. M., Rising, K., Kim, E. S., & Rapcsak, S. Z. (2010). A treatment sequence for phonological alexia/agraphia. *Journal of Speech, Language and Hearing Research, 53*(2), 450-468.

Behrmann, M., Shomstein, S. S., Black, S. E., & Barton, J. J. (2001). The eye movements of pure alexia patients during reading and nonreading tasks. *Neuropsychologia, 39,* 982-1002.

Beis, J. M., Keller, C., Morin, N., Bartolomeo, P., Bernati, T., Chokron, S., ... Azouvi, M. D. (2004). Right spatial neglect after left hemisphere stroke: Qualitative and quantitative study. *Neurology, 63*(9), 1600-1605.

Berteletti, I., Lucangeli, D., & Zorzi, M. (2012). Representation of numerical and non-numerical order in children. *Cognition, 124*(3), 304-313.

Beschin, N., Cisari, C., Cubelli, R., & Della Sala, S. (2014). Prose reading in neglect. *Brain and Cognition, 84,* 69-75.

Bressler-Richardson, E. (1996). *Cognitive reorganization: Practical math workbook.* Austin, TX: Pro-ed.

Cate, Y. and Richards, L. (2000). Relationship between performance on tests of basic visual functions and visual-perceptual processing in persons after brain injury. *American Journal of Occupational Therapy, 54*(3), 326-334.

Cherney, L. R. (2004). Aphasia, alexia and oral reading. *Topics in Stroke Rehabilitation, 11*(1), 22-36.

Cherney, L. R., Merbitz, C. T., & Grip, J. C. (1986). Efficacy of oral reading in aphasia treatment outcome. *Rehabilitation Literature, 47*(5-6), 112-118.

Cooper, J. & Jamal, N. (2012). Convergence insufficiency—a major review. *Optometry, 83*(4), 137-158.

Danan, M. (2004). Captioning and Subtitling: Undervalued language learning strategies. *Meta 491,* 67-77.

Dehaene, S. (2011). The massive impact of literacy on the brain and its consequences or education. *Human Neuroplasticity and Education, (Vatican City), 117,* 19-32.

Department of Veterans Affairs, Department of Defense. (2009). VA/DoD Clinical Practice Guidelines for Management of Concussion/Mild Traumatic Brain Injury (mTBI). *Journal of Rehabilitation Research and Development.* 46(6):CP1-68.

Devinsky, O. & D'Esposito, M. (2004). *Neurology of cognitive and behavioral disorders.* New York, NY: Oxford University Press.

Dusek, W. A., Pierscionek, B. K., & McClelland, J. F. (2011). An evaluation of clinical treatment of convergence insufficiency fort children with reading difficulties. *BMC Ophthalmology, 11,* 21. doi: 10.1186/1471-2415-11-21.

Edmans, J. & Lincoln, N. B. (1987). The frequency of perceptual deficits after stroke. *Clinical Rehabilitation, 52*(7), 266-270.

Fahle, M. & Greenlee, M. (2003). *The neuropsychology of vision.* New York, NY: Oxford University Press.

Flowers, D. L., Jones, K., Noble, K., VanMeter, J., Zeffiro, T. A., Wood, F. B., & Eden, G. F. (2004). Attention to single letters activates left extrastriate cortex. *Neuroimage, 21,* 829-839.

Gathercole, S. E. (1999). Cognitive approaches to the development of short-term memory. *Trends in Cognitive Sciences, 3*(11), 410-419.

Gathercole, S. E., Gauthier, L., Dehaut, F., & Joanette, Y. (1989). The Bells Test: A quantitative and qualitative test for visual neglect. *International Journal of Clinical Neuropsychology, 11,* 49-54.

Gianutsos, R. (1997). Vision rehabilitation following acquired brain injury. In M. Gentile (Ed.), *Functional Visual Behavior: A Therapist's Guide to Evaluation and Treatment Options.* Bethesda, MD: American Occupational Therapy Association, Inc.

Gillen, G. (2009). *Cognitive and perceptual rehabilitation: Optimizing function.* St. Louis, MO: Mosby Elsevier.

Goldman, M. & Goldman, S. (1988). Reading with closed-captioned TV. *Journal of Reading, 31,* 458-461.

Goldstein, K. & Gelb, A. (1918). Psychologishe Analysen hirnpathologischer Falle auf Grund von Untersuchungen Hirnverletzer. *Zeitschrift für die gesamte Neurologie und Psychiatrie, 41,* 1-42.

Goodwin, D. (2014). Homonymous hemianopia: Challenges and solutions. *Clinical Ophthalmology, 8,* 1919-1027.

Gordon-Salant, S., & Callahan, J. (2009). The benefits of hearing aids and closed captioning for television viewing by older adults with hearing loss. *Ear and Hearing, 30,* 458-465.

Grainger, J. & Holcomb, P. J. (2009). Watching the word go by: On the time-course of component processes in visual word recognition. *Language and Linguistics Compass, 3*(1), 128-156.

Greene, J. D. (2005). Apraxia, agnosias, and higher visual function abnormalities. *Journal of Neurology, Neurosurgery, and Psychiatry, 76*(Suppl. V), v25-v34.

Griffin, R. & Dumestre, J. (1993). An initial evaluation of the use of captioned television to improve the vocabulary and reading comprehension of Navy sailors. *Educational Technology, 22,* 193-296.

Hamilton, J. M. & Sanford, A. J. (1978). The symbolic distance effect for alphabetic order judgements: A subjective report and reaction time analysis. *Quarterly Journal of Experimental Psychology, 30,* 33-43.

Hillis, A.E. (2006). Rehabilitation of unilateral spatial neglect: New insights from magnetic resonance perfusion imaging. *Archives of Physical Medicine and Rehabilitation, 887*(12 Suppl.), S43-S49.

Hillis, A. E., Rapp, B., & Caramazza, A. (1999). When a rose is a rose in speech but a tulip in writing. *Cortex, 35,* 337-356.

Honig, B. (1996). *Teaching our children to read: The role of skills in a comprehensive reading program.* Thousand Oaks, CA: Corwin Press.

Jackson, G. R. & Owsley, C. (2003). Visual dysfunction, neurodegenerative diseases, and aging. *Neurologic Clinics of North America, 21,* 709-729.

James, K. H. & Gauthier, I. (2006). Letter processing automatically recruits a sensory-motor brain network. *Neuropsychologia, 44,* 2937-2949.

Jensema, C. (1996). Closed-captioned television: Presentation, speed, and vocabulary. *American Annals of the Deaf, 141,* 284-292.

Kaplan, E., Goodglass, H., & Weintraub, S. (2001). *Boston Naming Test* (2nd ed.). Philadelphia, PA: Lippincott, Williams, & Wilkins.

Kay, J., Lesser, R. & Coltheart, M. (1992). *PALPA: Psycholinguistic Assessments of Language Processing in Aphasia.* Hove, UK: Lawrence Erlbaum Associates.

Kemper, S. & McDowd, J. (2006). Eye movements of young and older adults while reading with distraction. *Psychology of Aging, 21,* 32-39.

Kerkhoff, G. (2000). Neurovisual rehabilitation: Recent developments and future directions. *Journal of Neurology, Neurosurgery & Psychiatry, 68,* 691-706.

Kerkhoff, G. & Schenk, T. (2012). Rehabilitation of neglect: an update. *Neuropsychologia, 50,* 10072-1079.

Kerkhoff, G., Keller, I., Ritter, V., & Marquardt, C. (2006). Repetitive optokinetic stimulation induces lasting recovery from visual neglect. *Restorative Neurology and Neuroscience, 24,* 357-369.

Kilpatrick, K. (1977). *Therapy guide for language and speech disorders, Vol. I: A selection of stimulus materials.* New York, NY: Visiting Nurse Service.

Kim, E. S. & Lemke, S. F. (2016). Behavioural and eye-movement outcomes in response to text-based reading treatment for acquired alexia. *Neurological Rehabilitation, 26*(1), 60-86.

Kim, E. S. & Russo, S. (2010). Multiple oral reading (MOR) treatment: Who is it for? *Contemporary Issues in Communication Science and Disorders, 37*, 58-68.

Kim, E. S., Rapcsak, S. Z., Anderson, S., & Beeson, P. M. (2011). Multimodal alexia: Neuropsychological mechanisms and implications for treatment. *Neuropsychologia, 49*, 3551-3562.

Kim, E. S., Rising, K., Rapcsak, S. Z., & Beeson, P. M. (2015). Treatment for alexia with agraphia following left ventral occipito-temporal damage: Strengthening orthographic representations common to reading and spelling. *Journal of Speech, Language and Hearing Research, 58*, 1521-1537.

Kinsbourne, M. & Warrington, E. K. (1962) A variety of reading disability associated with right hemisphere lesions. *Journal of Neurology, Neurosurgery & Psychiatry, 25*, 339-344.

Kleinman, J. T., Newhart, M., Davis, C., Heidler-Gary, J., Gottesman, R. F., & Hillis, A. E. (2007). Right hemispatial neglect: Frequency and characterization following acute left hemisphere stroke. *Brain and Cognition, 64*(1), 50-59.

Klingelhofer, J. & Conrad, B. (1984). Eye movements during reading in aphasics. *European Archives of Psychiatry and Neurological Sciences, 234*, 175-183.

Koskinen, P., Wilson, R., & Jensema, C. (1985). Closed-captioned television: A new tool for reading instruction. *Reading World, 24*, 1-7.

Koskinen, P., Knable, J., Markham, P., Jensema, C., & Kane, K. (1996). Captioned television and the vocabulary acquisition of adult second language. *Journal of Educational Technology Systems, 24*, 359-373.

Land, M. F. (2006). Eye movements and the control of actions in everyday life. *Progress in Retinal and Eye Research, 25*, 296-324.

Landis, T., Graves, R., Benson, F., & Hebben, N. (1982). Visual recognition through kinesthetic mediation. *Psychological Medicine, 12*, 515-531.

LaPointe, L. & Horner, J. (2006). *The Reading Comprehension Battery for Aphasia-2*. Austin, TX: Pro-Ed.

Leff, A. & Starrfelt, R. (2014). *Alexia: Diagnosis, treatment and theory*. London, UK: Springer.

Leff, A. P., Crewes, H., Plant, G. T., Scott, S. K., Kennard, C., & Wise, R. J. (2001). The functional anatomy of single-word reading in patients with hemianopic and pure alexia. *Brain, 124*, 510-521.

Likova, L. (2014). Learning-based cross-modal plasticity in the human brain: Insights from visual deprivation fMRI. *Journal of Advanced Brain Neuroimaging Topics in Health and Disease Methods and Applications*, 327-358. doi: 10.5772/58263.

Lott, S. N., Carney, A. S., Glezer, L. S., & Friedman, R. B. (2010). Overt use of tactile-kinesthetic strategy shifts to covert processing in rehabilitation of latter-by-letter reading. *Aphasiology, 24*(11), 1424-1442.

Margolis, N. W. (2011). Evaluation and treatment of visual field loss and visual-spatial neglect. In: P. S. Suter, & L. H. Harvey (Eds.), *Vision Rehabilitation: Multidisciplinary care of the patient following brain injury*. Boca Raton, Florida: CRC Press.

Markham, P. (1999). Captioned videotapes and second-language listening word recognition. *Foreign Language Annals, 32*(3), 321-328.

Martinoff, J. T., Martinoff, R., & Stokke, V. (1981). *Language rehabilitation: Auditory comprehension*. Austin, TX: Pro-ed.

Mayer, J. F. & Murray, L. L. (2002). Approaches to the treatment of alexia in chronic aphasia. *Aphasiology, 16*(7), 727-743.

McMartin Heeringa, H. (2002). *A manual for the treatment of acquired reading and writing disorders*. Ann Arbor, MI: SLP-Pathways.

Menichelli, A., Rapp, B., & Semenza, C. (2008). Allographic agraphia: A case study. *Cortex, 44*, 861-868.

Menichelli, A., Machetta, F., Zadini, A., & Semenza, C. (2012). Allographic agraphia for single letters. *Behavioural Neurology, 25*, 1-12.

Mozzo, M. & Caramazza, A. (1998). Varieties of pure alexia: The case of failure to access graphemic representations. *Cognitive Neuropsychology, 15*(1/2), 203-238.

Moyer, S. B. (1979). Rehabilitation of alexia: A case study. *Cortex, 15*, 139-144.

Myers, P. S. (1999). *Right hemisphere damage: Disorders of communication and cognition*. San Diego, CA: Singular Publishing Group.

Neggers, S. F. & Bekkering, H. (2001). Gaze anchoring to a pointing target is present during the entire pointing movement and is driven by a non-visual signal. *Journal of Neurophysiology, 86*, 961-970.

Ota, H., Fujii, T., Suzuki, K., Fukatsu, R., & Yamadori, A. (2011). Dissociation of body-centered and stimulus-centered representations in unilateral neglect. *Neurology, 57*, 2064-2069.

Pizzamiglio, L., Perani, D., Cappa, S. F., Vallar, G., Paolucci, S., Grassi, F., ... Ferruccio, F. (1998). Recovery of neglect after right hemisphere damage: H2(15)o Positron emission tomographic activation study. *Archives of Neurology, 55*, 561-568.

Powell, J. M. & Torgerson, G. (2011). Evaluation and treatment of vision and motor dysfunction following acquired brain injury from occupational therapy and neuro-optometry perspectives. In: P. S. Suter, & L. H. Harvey (Eds.), *Vision rehabilitation: Multidisciplinary care of the patient following brain injury* (pp. 356-396). Boca Raton, FL: CRC Press.

Purcell ,J. J., Turkeltaub, P. E., Eden, G. F., & Rapp, B. (2011). Examining the central and peripheral processes of written word production through meta-analysis. *Frontiers of Psychology, 2*, 1-16.

Purcell, J. J., Napoliello, E. M., & Eden, G. F. (2011a). A combined fMRI study of typed spelling and reading. *NeuroImage*, *55*, 750-762.

Rayner, K. (1979). Eye guidance in reading: Fixation locations within words. *Perception*, *8*(1), 21-30.

Rayner, K., Slattery, T. J., & Belanger, N. N. (2010). Eye movements and the perceptual span in older and younger readers. *Psychology and Aging*, *24*(3), 755-760.

Reicher, G. M. (1969). Perceptual recognition as a function of meaningfulness of stimulus material. *Journal of Experimental Psychology*, *81*, 274-280.

Reinhart, S., Schindler, I., & Kerkhoff, G. (2011). Optokinetic stimulation affects word omissions but not stimulus-centered reading errors in paragraph reading in neglect dyslexia. *Neuropsychologia*, *49*, 2728-2735.

Riley, J. (1996). *The teaching of reading. London,* UK: Paul Chapman Publishing.

Roeser, R. J., Valent, M., & Hosford-Dunn, H. (2007). *Audiology diagnosis* (2nd ed.). New York, NY: Thieme Medical Publishers, Inc.

Sanet, R. B. & Press, L. J. (2011). Spatial vision. In: P. S. Suter, & L. H. Harvey (Eds.), *Vision rehabilitation: Multidisciplinary care of the patient following brain injury* (pp. 77-151). Boca Raton, FL: CRC Press.

Scheiman, M. (2011). *Understanding and managing vision deficits: A guide for occupational therapists.* Thorofare, NJ: SLACK Incorporated.

Schmidt, M. & Haydu, M. (1992). The older hearing-impaired adult in the classroom: Real-Time closed captioning as a technological alternative to the oral lecture. *Educational Gerontology*, *18*, 273-276.

Sinanovi, O., Mrkonji, S., Vidovi, M., & Imamovi, K. (2011). Post-stroke language disorders. *Acta Clinica Croatica*, *50*(1), 79-94.

Spitzyna, G. A., Wise, R. J., McDonald, S. A., Plant, G. T., Kidd, D., Crewes, H., & Leff, A. P. (2007). Optokinetic therapy improves text reading in patients with hemianopic alexia. *Neurology*, *68*, 1922-1930.

Spreen, O. & Strauss, E. (1998). *A compendium of neuropsychological tests: Administration, norms, and commentary* (2nd ed.). New York, NY: Oxford University Press.

Tannen, B. M. & Ciuffreda, K. J. (2007). A proposed addition to the standard protocol for the Visagraph II™ Eye movement recording system. *Journal of Behavioral Optometry*, *18*(6), 143-147.

Taylor, S. E. (2000). *Visagraph II Eye-Movement Recording System.* Huntingon, NY: Taylor Associates/Communications, Inc.

Teasell, R., Salter, K., Cotoi, A., Brar, J., & Donais, J. (2016). Perceptual disorders. *Evidence-Based Review of Stroke Rehabilitation*, 1-66.

Townend, B. S., Sturm, J. W., Petsoglou, C., O'Leary B., Whyte, S., & Crimmins, D. (2007). Perimetric homonymous visual field loss post-stroke. *Journal of Clinical Neuroscience*, *14*(8), 754-756.

Tse, P., Baumgartner, F., & Greenlee, M. (2010). Event-related functional MRI of cortical activity evoked by microsaccades, small visually-guided saccades, and eyblinks in human visual cortex. *Neuroimage*, *49*(1), 805-816.

VaDoD Clinical Practice Guidelines for the Management of Stroke Rehabilitation (2010). Version 2.0, Section 4.5, 22. Assessment of Sensory Impairment: Touch, Vision, Hearing. Retrieved from https://www.rehab.research.va.gov/jour/10/479/pdf/VADODcliniaclGuidelines479.pdf Accessed on December 17, 2018.

Vanderplank, R. (1988). The value of teletext subtitles in language learning. *ELT Journal*, *42*(4), 272-281.

West, J. (2009). Recovery of functional reading in a client with alexia. ASHA Convention: Poster Session *1823*, 202.

Wilson, B. A. & Evans, J. J. (1996). Error-free learning in the rehabilitation of people with memory impairments. *Journal of Head Trauma Rehabilitation*, *11*(2), 54-64.

Withrow F. (1994). The walls come tumbling down! *American Annals of the Deaf*, *139*, 18-21.

Wolf, M. (2007). *Proust and the squid: The story and science of the reading brain.* New York, NY: HarperCollins, Publishers.

Wood, J. & McLemore, B. (2001). Critical components in early literacy—Knowledge of the letters of the alphabet and phonics instruction. *The Florida Reading Quarterly*, *38*(2), 1-8.

Woodhead, Z.V.J., Ong, Y.-H., & Leff, A.P. (2015). Web-based therapy for hemianopic alexia is syndrome-specific. *BMJ Innovations*, 1:88-95.

Zihl, J. (1995). Eye movement patterns in hemianopic dyslexia. *Brain*, *118*, 891-912.

Zihl, J. (2000). *Neuropsychological rehabilitation: A modular handbook, rehabilitation of visual disorders after brain injury.* London, UK: Psychological Press Ltd.

Glossary

A

- **Accommodation reflex:** contraction of the ciliary muscle resulting in rounding of the lens, contraction of the pupil, and convergence of the eyes when there is accommodation for near vision. The adjustment in the ocular lens that changes refractive power in order to focus the image of an object on the retina for near and far vision. It is measured in diopters and normally diminishes with age.
- **Achromatopsia:** loss of color vision due to lesions in the basal temporal occipital cortex.
- **Agnosia:** the inability to recognize common objects despite an intact visual system; attributed to lesions of the ventral (central) visual pathway.
- **Akinetopsia:** the inability to perceive motion; moving objects appear to jump from one location to another.

B

- **Balint syndrome:** acquired inability to perceive the visual field as a whole, which results in the varied perception and recognition of only parts of the visual field; results from bilateral parietal or parietal-occipital lesions; involves three components variously described as: a) visual inattention, impaired gaze shifting, and impaired visually-guided reaching; or b) oculomotor apraxia or psychic paralysis of gaze, spatial restriction of attention, and optic ataxia; characterized by the inability to shift one's gaze to a new stimulus to reach or to point. Gaze appears to wander aimlessly and targets are located by chance; impaired perception of the position and distance of objects in relation to the viewer. Individuals with this syndrome may make statements such as "I can see the clock but I don't know where it is." These individuals are unable to perform saccadic shifts, including right-to-left return sweep movements in order to read sentences and paragraphs.
- **Binocular disparity:** the perceived difference in the image presented to each eye that occurs because our eyes are offset in the horizontal plane; each eye has a slightly different view.

McMartin Heeringa, H. *The Visual Brain and Peripheral Reading and Writing Disorders: A Guide to Visual System Dysfunction for Speech-Language Pathologists.* (pp. 77-82). © 2019 Taylor & Francis Group.

- **Binocular vision:** visual sensation that occurs when the two offset images presented to each eye are fused together at the cortical level.
- **Broca's aphasia:** non-fluent aphasia resulting from lesions of the third frontal convolution of the left hemisphere; characterized by anomia, paraphasic substitution errors, agrammatism; impaired verbal repetition and written formulation; auditory comprehension is impaired to a lesser degree.

C

- **Central language processes:** the sublexical components such as phonological processing (letter-sound/sound-letter conversion) and the (working memory component of oral and written spelling).
- **Closed captions:** strings of text presented on the television screen that mimic or closely match audio content; typical presentation duration is six seconds for two lines of text.
- **Cones:** photoreceptor cells that respond to bright light and color stimulation of the fovea, in the central retina.
- **Conjugate gaze:** coordinated movement of the eyes in the same direction; tested in all directions of gaze.
- **Convergence:** rotation of the eyes toward midline to view objects at near distances; the closer the object the greater the degree of convergence.

D

- **Depth perception:** the ability to judge the relative distance of one object to another (allocentric perspective), and the distance from an object to oneself (egocentric perspective); information on binocular disparity is combined with monocular cues such as texture, relative size, and linear perspective to achieve the perception of depth; this binocular information is integrated through the corpus callossum.
- **Diplopia:** the impression of duplicated images or objects; may occur in the entire field of vision, or when gazing in a particular direction; occurs following stroke, traumatic brain injury, brain tumor or other neurological disorder; attributed to impaired eye alignment.

F

- **Field of vision:** see Useful Field of View.
- **Fixation:** the static horizontal and vertical eye position between the end of one saccade and the start of the next saccade when scanning a series of stationary objects such as words; during reading, fixation occurs to the left of the middle of words.
- **Fovea:** portion of the central retina that contains only cone cells, the photoreceptors for daylight vision; the fovea represents the central one degree of vision.

G

- **Gaze apraxia:** inability to shift one's gaze from one location to another; seen in Balint syndrome following damage to bilateral parietal lobes.
- **Global alexia:** the reader is able to identify pictures but unable to identify most or all letters and words; persons with global alexia are unable to use the letter-by-letter reading strategy.
- **Graphemes:** abstract letter representations (not letter names or shapes).
- **Graphemic buffer:** the working memory component of oral and written spelling; letters and words are retrieved from the orthographic lexicon (long-term memory for words) and held in the graphemic buffer until the word is spelled.

- **Graphic features:** capital or lower case; print or cursive; single or doubled letters, e.g. lesson; syllable structure; consonant-vowel status.

H

- **Hemianopia:** loss of vision in the right or left half of the visual field.

L

- **Left hemifield:** area of the visual field that provides input to the left nasal retina and the right temporal retina; input to the left nasal retina crosses over at the optic chiasm to the right hemisphere; input to the right temporal retina provides direct input to the right hemisphere.
- **Letter-by-Letter reading:** the act of decoding and naming letters one by one in order to decipher words. This is a compensatory reading strategy and a symptom of pure alexia.

M

- **Macropsia:** visual condition in which objects look larger than they really are; caused by lesions in the basal temporal occipital cortex.
- **Micropsia:** visual condition in which objects look smaller than they really are; caused by lesions in the basal temporal occipital cortex.
- **Microsaccades:** fast, conjugate involuntary eye movements that recenter images on the central retina. Microsaccades repeatedly stimulate retinal ganglia to fire during sustained fixation, and are important to reading.

N

- **Near visual acuity:** the extent to which an individual is able to see and identify objects or words within an arm's length.
- **Nystagmus:** involuntary oscillation of the eyeball that may be horizontal, vertical, torsional or mixed.

O

- **O.D.:** oculus dexter, or right eye.
- **O.D.:** Doctor of Optometry
- **Ophthalmoplegia:** paralysis of the ocular muscles; O.externa is paralysis of the extraocular muscles; O.interna is paralysis of the iris and ciliary muscle.
- **Optic ataxia:** a disorder of central visually guided movement resulting from bilateral damage to the parietal lobes; occurs in Balint syndrome.
- **Optic chiasm:** the x-shaped crossing of the optic nerve fibers; fibers originating in the inner half of the retina (nasal retina) cross over to the contralateral hemisphere at the optic chiasm. This aids binocular vision.
- **Optic disk:** blind spot, the portion of the retina where the optic nerve enters.
- **Optic nerve:** the second cranial nerve (II) that carries visual impulses from the retina, through the optic chiasm and optic tract to the thalamus.
- **Optic radiation:** a system of fibers that extend from the lateral geniculate body of the thalamus through the sublenticular portion of the internal capsule to the calcarine occipital cortex (striate cortex).
- **Optic tract:** fibers extending from the optic nerve beyond the optic chiasm; the majority of these fibers terminate in the lateral geniculate body (nucleus) of the thalamus; a portion of these fibers extend to the superior colliculus of the midbrain.

- **Optokinetic reflex:** a quick, reflexive saccade that is triggered in the reverse direction, when the eyes follow a moving object; allows the viewer to keep the head stable when viewing moving objects.
- **Optokinetic stimulation:** a graphic display of text moving toward the left; this type of stimulation triggers a quick reflexive eye movement toward the right (optokinetic reflex). An example of this type of graphic display is news headlines that scroll at the bottom of a TV screen.
- **Orthographic representation:** the way in which sounds are represented by written symbols; phoneme-grapheme mapping. Knowledge of orthography includes knowing, for example, that the bigram "ph" sounds like /f/.
- **Orthographic buffer:** the working memory component for writing and typing. Words are retrieved from long-term memory and held briefly in the orthographic buffer or "visuospatial sketchpad" until they are converted to letter names (in oral spelling), and graphemes (in writing). It is hypothesized that the primary visual cortex (V1) is the site of the visuospatial sketchpad (Likova, 2014).
- **Orthographic lexicon:** the long-term storage of all the words an individual knows.
- **Orthoptics:** treatment of deficits of binocular visual function or of the muscles controlling movement of the eyes.
- **O.S.:** oculus sinister, or left eye.

P

- **Palinopsia:** also called visual perseveration, where the individual continues to see details of a visual scene or of print even after having looked away from it; occurs in Charles Bonnet syndrome; may result from focal occipital or occipitoparietal lesions, or from disease of the optic nerve or the eye (Pomeranz et al, 2000); also associated with LSD or ecstasy (Kawasaki & Purvin, 1996; McGuire et al, 1994) .
- **Peripheral dyslexia:** reading disorders due to impairment in the processing of visual stimuli such as letters and words.
- **Phoneme-Grapheme conversion system:** this system consists of two processes for spelling unfamiliar words (nonwords or pseudowords): 1) phonological organization of auditory input into smaller units (i.e. syllables, or phonemes); and 2) phoneme-grapheme assignment.
- **Phonological awareness:** the ability to hear the sounds that form words in spoken language; includes recognizing rhyming words, determining whether a word begins and ends with the same sound, and being able to separate words into their individual sounds.
- **Prism:** in relation to vision therapy, a wedge of transparent material that deviates light rays without changing their focus. Base-in prism (BI) displaces the visual space outward and expands visual space volume. Base-out prism (BO) displaces the visual space inward.
- **Prosopagnosia:** impaired facial recognition caused by damage to the right medial temporal lobe.
- **Pure alexia (alexia without agraphia):** acquired peripheral reading disorder associated with posterior circulation strokes. The reader with pure alexia is unable to identify letters and/or words. Use of the letter-by-letter reading strategy is a hallmark of pure alexia. A high percentage of cases of pure alexia have a right homonymous visual field deficit. These clients are typically not aphasic as auditory comprehension, verbal expression and writing are generally intact. Pure alexics are unable to read their own writing.

Q

- **Quadrantanopia:** loss of vision in one quarter of the visual field; in right quadrantanopia there is a right upper field deficit consistently associated with lesions of the lower lip of the left primary visual cortex (V1). In left quadrantanopia there is a left upper field deficit consistently associated with lesions of the lower lip of the right primary visual cortex (V1).

R

- **Reading saccades:** small-scale, eye movements that alternate with gaze fixations during reading;
- **Refractive power:** the degree to which a transparent body (such as the cornea, aqueous humor, crystalline lens, or vitreous body) deflects a ray of light from a straight path.
- **Retina:** the light-sensitive portion of the eye which extends from the optic disk to the border of the pupil; each portion of the retina including the fovea (central retina) is represented in the primary visual cortex (V1).
- **Rods:** retinal photoreceptor cells which respond to dim or low light; rods are concentrated in the peripheral retina.

S

- **Scanning:** the ability to perform successive saccades in order to read, locate items in a drawer, or to locate distant objects within the environment.
- **Scotoma:** partial area of blindness in the visual field; lesions in the upper left lip of area V1 (striate cortex) will predictably cause blindness in the contralateral lower right field of view. Similarly, lesions in the lower right lip of area V1 will predictably cause blindnes in the contralateral upper left field of view.
- **Simultanagnosia:** the inability to recognize or attend to more than one object in the field of view at a time.
- **Stereognosis:** the ability to recognize the form of solid objects by touch.
- **Stereopsis:** the ability to perceive depth because of minor differences in the offset image processed by each eye; eye teaming ability is a foundation skill for stereopsis.
- **Striate cortex:** (V1) or primary visual cortex; nerve cells in V1 detect lines and shapes in a specific manner. The right striate cortex receives input from the right (ipsilateral) temporal retina, and from the left (contralateral) nasal retina to detect objects and events in the left visual field. The left striate cortex receives in put from the left (ipsilateral) temporal retina and from the right (contralateral) nasal retina to detect objects and events in the right visual field.
- **Sublexical:** refers to knowledge of language that is manifest prior to word recognition e.g., knowledge of sound-letter correspondence (phonological spelling); knowing that /k/ can be written as "k" or "K," "c" or "C," "q" or "Q."

T

- **Tracking:** the ability to follow moving objects such as balls, people, and autos smoothly and accurately using both eyes.

U

- **Useful field of view (UFOV):** this is the area within which the viewer can take in information without any head or eye movement. With regard to reading, the useful field of view, also called the "visual span," is the number of letters and words that can be grouped and analyzed within one fixation.

V

- **Ventral stream:** a visual pathway that connects the occipital and temporal lobes; detects fine details of objects, letters and words; necessary for reading and the recognition of forms.
- **Visual acuity:** in reference to visual clarity; measured using the Snellen Chart, and is reported as 20/20, 20/40, etc. "20/20 vision" means that an individual sees from a distance of 20 feet what the normal eye is able to see at that distance. Whereas, "20/40 vision" means that an individual sees at 40 feet what the normal eye would see at 20 feet.
- **Visual agnosia:** the inability to integrate lines and edges in order to construct simple and/or complex forms. Persons with visual agnosia may be able to see and copy the simplest elements of a design without identifying the whole.
- **Visual cortex:** located in the occipital lobe; includes area V1 which is referred to as the striate cortex or primary visual cortex, and the prestriate cortex.
- **Visual field:** the normal range of central and peripheral vision; often diminished in neurological disease due to head injury and stroke.
- **Visuospatial sketchpad:** see Orthographic buffer.

W

- **Wernicke's aphasia:** language impairment characterized by significant impairment in auditory comprehension with intact auditory acuity; impaired word and sentence repetition; and fluent speech marked by paraphasic errors; occurs with lesions to superior temporal convolution of the left hemisphere.
- **Word length effect:** the observation that persons who use a letter-by-letter reading strategy take longer to read longer words than shorter words.

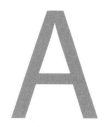

Test Instruments for the Assessment of Peripheral Reading and Writing Disorders

TABLE A-1	
ARIZONA BATTERY FOR READING AND SPELLING	
MEASURES OF READING	**MEASURES OF WRITING**
Reading List 1: Regular and irregular, high- and low-frequency words (40 words)	Spelling List 1: Same as Reading List 1 but written to dictation
Reading List 2: Regular and irregular, high- and low-frequency words (40 words)	Spelling List 2: Same as Reading List 2 but written to dictation
Nonwords Reading List: (20 words)	Nonwords Spelling List: Same as Nonwords Reading List but written to dictation

TABLE A-2	
ASSESSMENT OF LANGUAGE-RELATED FUNCTIONAL ACTIVITIES	
MEASURES OF READING	**MEASURES OF WRITING**
• Telling time (reading clock face) • Counting money (discriminating coins and bills) • Solving daily math problems (option to read story problems or listen to them) • Reading instructions • Reading medication labels	• Addressing an envelope • Writing a check and balancing a checkbook register • Writing phone messages • Reading a bill

McMartin Heeringa, H. *The Visual Brain and Peripheral Reading and Writing Disorders: A Guide to Visual System Dysfunction for Speech–Language Pathologists.* (pp. 83-86).

TABLE A-3
BOSTON DIAGNOSTIC APHASIA EXAMINATION

MEASURES OF READING	MEASURES OF WRITING
• Basic symbol recognition • Number matching • Arabic numbers matched to dot patterns • Roman numbers matched to Arabic numbers • Word identification: Picture-word match and lexical decision (i.e., discriminating real words from nonwords) • Phonics: Match homophones (i.e., vowel discrimination task) and pseudohomophones (i.e., advanced phonic analysis) • Derivational and grammatical morphology matching (i.e., match spoken word to one of four written words) • Bound grammatical morphemes • Derivational morphemes • Oral reading of words • Oral reading of sentences with comprehension • Comprehension: Sentence completion, sentences, and paragraphs	• Writing mechanics: Signature, printed name, dictated letters (5 stimuli), abbreviations, copy sentence (cursive/print), full alphabet, numbers 1 through 10, and dictated numbers (5 stimuli) • Dictated words: Primer-level dictation (5 stimuli), spelling to dictation (10 stimuli) • Phonics, common irregular forms • Uncommon irregularities and nonsense words • Oral spelling • Written picture naming: Objects, actions, and animals • Cognitive/grammatical influences on written word • Retrieval: Part of speech effects and dictated functor-loaded sentences • Narrative writing: Cookie theft picture

TABLE A-4	
WESTERN APHASIA BATTERY	
MEASURES OF READING	**MEASURES OF WRITING**
• Comprehension of sentences • Reading commands • Written word–object choice matching • Written word–picture choice matching • Spoken word–written word choice matching • Picture–written word choice matching • Letter discrimination • Spelled word recognition • Spelling • Reading irregular words • Reading nonwords	• Writing upon request • Writing output • Writing to dictation • Writing dictated words • Alphabet and numbers • Dictated letters and numbers • Copying a sentence • Writing irregular words to dictation • Writing nonwords to dictation

TABLE A-5
READING COMPREHENSION BATTERY FOR APHASIA-2: SELECTED SUBTESTS
Word-picture matching subtests: Visual, auditory, semantic Functional reading Sentence-picture matching Paragraph-picture matching
RCBA-2 SUPPLEMENTAL PICTURE BOOK
• Letter discrimination (x40): The reader determines if two printed uppercase letters are the same. • Letter naming: 12 letters are presented in 2 rows at either the left or right of midline. • Letter recognition: A field of 44 uppercase printed letters are presented in random order. The reader points to the letter named by the clinician. • Lexical decision (x20): A field of three lowercase, printed words is presented in a list. The reader is instructed to point to the one word that is a real word. • Semantic categorization (x40): Two words are presented; one is a category name in uppercase letters, the other is an object name in lowercase print. The reader is instructed to state whether the two words belong together (i.e., are semantically related). • Oral reading—words (x30): Five lowercase printed words presented in list form. The reader is instructed to read each word aloud. • Oral reading—sentences (x30): Five sentences in lowercase print are presented in list form. The reader is instructed to read each sentence aloud.

TABLE A-6
SELECTED SUBTESTS OF THE PSYCHOLINGUISTIC ASSESSMENTS OF LANGUAGE PROCESSING ABILITIES

- Letter discrimination: Mirror reversal, upper-lower case match, lower-upper case match, words and nonwords
- Letter naming and sound-letter correspondence
- Spoken letter–written letter matching
- Visual lexicon decision: Legality, imageability x frequency, morphological endings, regularity
- Homophone decision
- Oral reading: Letter length, syllable length, imageability x frequency, grammatical class, grammatical class x imageability
- Morphological endings
- Oral reading: Regularity, nonwords, sentences
- Homophone definition x regularity
- Spelling to dictation: Letter length, imageability x frequency, grammatical class, grammatical class x imageability, morphological endings, regularity, nonwords, disambiguated homophones

Criteria for Viewer-Centered, Stimulus-Centered, and Object-Centered Neglect

McMartin Heeringa, H. *The Visual Brain and Peripheral Reading and Writing Disorders: A Guide to Visual System Dysfunction for Speech–Language Pathologists*. (pp. 87–88).
© 2019 Taylor & Francis Group.

TABLE B-1		
CRITERIA FOR IMPAIRMENT		
VIEWER-CENTERED NEGLECT	**OBJECT-CENTERED NEGLECT**	**STIMULUS-CENTERED NEGLECT**
Significantly more errors on stimulus presentations in the left body field vs. the right body field on at least one of the following tasks: • Line cancellation • Gaps • Bells test • Line bisection	Significantly more errors on the contralesional side vs. the ipsilateral side of the canonical representation of words in the vertical word reading task.	Significantly more errors on the left vs. the right side of the page on at least one of the following tasks, presented both at midline of the patient's body and in at least one of the other body fields (left or right): • Line cancellation • Bells test
And/or significantly more errors on the left vs. the right side of the page on at least one of these tasks administered at midline: • Ogden scene • Gap detection task • Passage reading	And/or significantly more errors on the contralesional side vs. the ipsilesional side of words in single word reading and in mirror-reversed word reading. And/or significantly more errors on the contralesional side vs. the ipsilesional side of words in recognition of oral spelling (i.e., clinician spells word aloud and client says the word).	And/or significantly more errors on the left side of the stimulus vs. the right side of the stimulus on at least one of the following tasks: • Ogden scene: Errors on left side of objects in scene vs. right side of objects in scene • Gap detection task: Fails to detect gap on left side of circle vs. right side of circle • Sentence reading: Errors on left side of word vs. right side of word
Source: Hillis, A.R. (2006). Neurobiology of Unilateral Spatial Neglect. *The Neuroscientist, 12,* 2 (pp. 153-163).		

C

Suggested Apps and Online Exercises for the Treatment of Acquired Reading and Writing Disorders

TABLE C-1

SUGGESTED APPS AND ONLINE EXERCISES FOR THE TREATMENT OF ACQUIRED READING AND WRITING DISORDERS

App	Modality/ Mode	Letter Recognition	Word Recognition	Written Spelling	Number Recognition	
Build-A-Word Express www.atreks.com		X	X			
Lingraphica TalkPath	Writing	X	X	X		
TACTUS Therapy www.tactustherapy.com	Writing	X	X	X		
Tracing Letters, Cursive Writing, and Cursive Words (Horizon Business, Inc.)	Writing	X				
Assistive Express App (AAC App) (Kiat Ng)	Writing Phrases			X		
Auditory ProcessingStudio (Virtual Speech Center, Inc.) Focuses attention to beginning, middle and end of words.	Auditory Discrimination/ Phonological Awareness/ Auditory Closure					
Auditory Concentration Memory Game www.manythings.org	Hearing					
Phonics Genius www.alligatorapps.com Focuses attention to beginning, middle and end of words.	Play Mode • Learning Words Only • Listening					
Optokinetic Stimulation (OKS) www.eyecanlearn.com (TimeSquare Scrolling Text)	Scanning		X			
Number Line, Number ID, Line 'em Up www.livecode.com					X	
Number Grid www.SmallerGames.net					X	

Scanning	Attention to Beginning, Middle, and End of Words	Speech Discrimination	Memory for Sounds in Words	Written Formulation	Motor Planning for Writing
					X
				X	
	X		X		
		X			
X	X		X		
X					
X					
X					

Keyboarding Exercise
Combining Motor Function with a Visual Language Exercise

GOALS

- Increase range of eye movements in context of typing/written spelling task.
- Improve letter recognition for written spelling.
- Evaluate use of typing as a compensatory skill for written expression.

Note: Consult with occupational therapist regarding upper extremity function relating to keyboarding.

Step 1.

Orient the client to the computer monitor, pointing out each corner. Instruct the client to trace the edges of the computer monitor (lower left corner to upper left corner; upper right corner to lower right corner) with his or her finger.

Step 2.

Show the client how to grasp the computer mouse. Place the softer side of Velcro strips on either side of the mouse where the client will grip it with thumb and middle fingers.

Step 3.

Draw the client's attention to the cursor. Show the client how to wiggle the mouse and ask him or her to visually locate the wiggling cursor. Show him or her how to make small movements with the mouse rather than larger, sweeping movements when trying to locate the cursor. Cue the client to use his or her eyes to guide hand-mouse movements.

McMartin Heeringa, H. *The Visual Brain and Peripheral Reading and Writing Disorders: A Guide to Visual System Dysfunction for Speech–Language Pathologists.* (pp. 93–94).
© 2019 Taylor & Francis Group.

Step 4.

Set small goals:
- Visually locate the cursor with verbal and gestural cues.
- Visually locate the cursor while wiggling the mouse.
- Place the cursor on a target (e.g., internet icon or large font block letter you have placed on a blank Microsoft Word document).
- Left click mouse without moving it from the letter or icon target.
- Move mouse along line of print to guide eyes in a left-to-right scanning pattern.

Step 5.

Orient the client to the computer keyboard:
- "With your left pointer finger, point to 'W' (clinician demonstrates) and with your right pointer finger, point to 'O' (clinician demonstrates)."
- Instruct the client to type letter pairs, with the left hand, right hand, and bimanually, then to type three-letter words. Provide verbal and gestural cues and physical assist as needed (see the following).

Left hand: WE, AS, AT, AD, BE, EX, FA
Right hand: UP, OH, ON, MY, MO, HI, NO
Left and right hands: TO, OR, IS, IT, AN, GO, YA
Left hand: WAS, WET, SEW, DEW, CAR, CAT, GET, RED, SET, FAR
Right hand: POP, MOP, PIN, LIP, HIP, HIM, HOP, INK, HOP, JOY
Left and right hands : TIM, ORE, PIT, JOB, LIT, HOT, NOT, KEY, THE, FRY
Left hand: REST, WEST, DATE, GATE, GAVE, EVER, GREW, REST, FADE
Right hand: PUMP, JUMP, LINK, MINK, HUMP, PUMP, PLUM, HULK, PINK
Left and right hands: HIRE, LIAR, LIKE, WENT, WIND, GONE, MINT, TRUE, HINT
Left hand: WARES, SWEAR, TEARS, CARES, GREAT, BRAVE, CREST
Right hand: PLUMP, MILLY, LUMPY, NINNY, JIMMY, JUMPY, MILKY
Left and right hands: BUNNY, HOUSE, PENNY, WORTH, GROWN, ABOUT, PEARL

1. TIM WANTED TO TRY HIS HAND AT GOLF.
2. MARY JUMPED ACROSS THE CHALK LINE.
3. WHEN DO YOU WANT TO EAT DINNER?
4. I WALKED THE DOG WHEN WE GOT HOME.
5. THE WIND BLEW HARD ALL NIGHT LONG.
6. THE MONEY HAS ALL BEEN SPENT.
7. TELL ME ABOUT YOUR VACATION.
8. THEIR CHILDREN ARE ALL GROWN.
9. MY BROTHER HIRED A MECHANIC.
10. I DON'T EVEN KNOW YOUR NAME.

Visual System Dysfunction in Progressive Neurological Disorders

In progressive neurological disease, visual deficits vary greatly depending upon the site and extent of lesions and may help with differential diagnosis based on distinct patterns of deficits in visual spatial processing (Possin, 2010). Appendix E provides a brief overview of the visual symptoms associated with a subset of progressive neurological disorders. Addressing object- and space-centered visual impairments in the dementias is difficult because performance on visual tasks is negatively impacted by dysexecutive syndrome, or *frontal lobe impairment*, including impairments in attention, switching perceptual sets/task switching, and working memory.

Multiple Sclerosis

Multiple sclerosis is a progressive neurological disorder caused by demyelination of multifocal areas of white matter in the central nervous system. It is characterized by motor weakness, fatigue, and sensory impairment. Initial symptoms occur between 25 and 30 years of age (Mort & Kennard, 2000). The incidence of multiple sclerosis in the United States is reported to be in the area of 1/100,000 people. Symptoms of visual involvement include nystagmus and impaired voluntary gaze impacting saccades and smooth pursuits, and diplopia (Barnes & McDonald, 1992). Bhatti et al. (2003) report that third nerve involvement caused enlarged pupil and ptosis of the eyelid in one subject with multiple sclerosis.

Myasthenia Gravis

Myasthenia gravis is an acquired autoimmune disorder. It is characterized by weakness of the skeletal muscles and patients are easily fatigued with exertion. Visual symptoms occur in most persons with myasthenia gravis, including blurring, diplopia (i.e., double vision) that fluctuates,

McMartin Heeringa, H. *The Visual Brain and Peripheral Reading and Writing Disorders: A Guide to Visual System Dysfunction for Speech–Language Pathologists.* (pp. 95-99).

nystagmus on lateral gaze due to ocular-motor weakness, and eyelid weakness brought on by exertion that results in ptosis (Roh, Lee, & Yoon, 2011). The ptosis is worsened with sustained upward gaze.

HUNTINGTON'S DISEASE

Huntington's disease (HD) is an inherited, progressive, autosomal dominant, neurological disorder characterized by abnormal, abrupt, involuntary movements that impact motor speech, swallowing, gait, and posture. Neurons of the globus pallidus, substantia nigra, ventral anterior nucleus of the thalamus, cerebellar dentate nucleus, brainstem, and spinal cord may also be affected (Heathfield, 1973; Lauterbach et al., 1998). HD affects approximately 4.1 to 7.5/100,000 people, with age at onset between 35 to 50 years. Symptoms associated with HD include movement disorders (e.g, chorea, dystonia) or Parkinsonism. Visual symptoms include deficits in voluntary eye movements with loss of rapid eye movements (i.e., saccades), square wave jerks (i.e., spontaneous movement of the eyes away from and back toward a fixated target), inability to suppress reflexive saccades when the eyes are fixated on a target, slow voluntary saccadic movements, and typically normal smooth pursuits (Mort & Kennard, 2000). As the disease progresses, visuospatial abilities may diminish (Gillen, 2009).

PARKINSON'S DISEASE

Parkinson's disease is a progressive movement disorder caused by the loss of dopaminergic neurons in the basal ganglia. It is the most common movement disorder with incidence of 50,000 Americans diagnosed each year (NINDS, 2018). Age at onset is between 55 to 65 years (Daniels, 2006). Causes of Parkinson's disease include neurodegenerative diseases, such as idiopathic Parkinson's disease, progressive supranuclear palsy, multiple system atrophy, corticobasal ganglionic degeneration, infarction of the basal ganglia due to chronic hypertension, and Wilson's disease (Mort & Kennard, 2000). Oculomotor features of Parkinson's include reduced blink rate, square wave jerks (see Huntington's disease), impaired smooth pursuits, reduction in the length of voluntary saccades, limitation in upward gaze, impaired convergence, and apraxia of eyelid opening or closing, reduced visual attention, problems perceiving structures from motion, reduced visual memory, reading comprehension deficits, and problems with perception of faces and objects (Jackson & Owsley, 2003). Visuospatial impairment is also noted in some cases of Parkinson's disease (Gillen, 2009; Possin, 2010).

DEMENTIA

There are several different types of dementia, defined by the location and nature of associated lesions, and the level and type of neurological dysfunction and disease progression. Within each category of dementia, visual motor and visual sensory systems may be affected differently.

Progressive Supranuclear Palsy

Progressive supranuclear palsy (PSP), a variant of frontotemporal dementia, is a neurodegenerative disease that impairs posture, balance, cognition, and oculomotor function. PSP involves the basal ganglia, brainstem, midbrain, and frontal lobes. It is characterized by pseudobulbar palsy, axial rigidity, and dementia. Dysarthria and dysphagia are noted early. Slow and shortened saccades are typically followed by a vertical gaze palsy (i.e., vertical ophthalmoplegia). Persons with PSP may also develop difficulty with horizontal gaze. Later signs include slower opening and closing of the eyes (Rehmann, 2000). There is preservation of visual spatial cognition and visual construction abilities but more marked deficits in higher-level spatial attention (Possin, 2010). In the U.S. population, the prevalence of PSP is approximately 1.39/100,000 people. Typical onset is between the ages of 50 to 60 years. PSP has also been found to affect 4% to 6% of persons with Parkinson's disease. In a study of 24 patients with PSP (Globe, Dais, Schoenberg, & Duvoisin, 1988), 13% of subjects had visual symptoms including diplopia, blurred vision, burning eyes, and light sensitivity. Persons with PSP will have difficulty with formal tests that require vertical saccades, such as the number-location subtest of the Visual Object Space Perception Battery (Warrington & James, 1991).

Alzheimer's Disease

Alzheimer's disease is the most common form of dementia and is characterized by both cognitive dysfunction and visual system impairments. Visual impairments have been found to be predictive of cognitive impairment in persons with Alzheimer's disease (Cronin-Golomb, Corkin, & Growdonn , 1995). Jackson and Owsley (2003) reviewed the literature on visual system dysfunction in the aging population with Alzheimer's disease and found that the visual association areas show more evidence of neurodegenerative changes. Deficits in visual attention, visual memory, spatial localization, and recognition of complex patterns were reported. Difficulty with visual discrimination and recognition of letters, objects, and faces were also noted. Rizzo, Anderson, Dawson, and Nawrot (2000) investigated the relationship between cognitive decline and impairment in the ventral and dorsal visual pathways in older subjects with and without Alzheimer's disease. The authors examined useful field of view (UFOV) as it relates to processing speed and the ability to perform visual divided attention and selective attention tasks. The UFOV is the area within which the viewer can take in information without any head or eye movement. Rizzo et al (2000) found a strong, positive correlation between UFOV and these measures of cognition. Lesions of the posterior parietal or inferior temporal cortex have been associated with a decrease in depth perception in persons with Alzheimer's disease (Mittenberg, Malloy, Petrick, & Knee, 1994). When there is posterior cortical atrophy in bilateral superior parietooccipital cortex, Alzheimer's disease subjects display symptoms of Balint syndrome (a spatial perceptual disorder), including simultanagnosia, optic ataxia, and oculomotor apraxia (Greene, 2005; Perez, Runkel, & Lachmann, 1996). Agraphia in the form of peripheral writing disorders (e.g., problems with written letter formation, letter case selection [upper- vs. lowercase], and cursive vs. print writing) are more evident as Alzheimer's disease progresses (Platel et al., 1993).

Posterior Cortical Atrophy

Posterior cortical atrophy (PCA) is a neurodegenerative syndrome (Wilson et al., 2013) and considered by some to be a variant of Alzheimer's disease (Tsai, Teng, Liu, & Menendez, 2011). It is associated with neurofibrillary tangles, senile plaques, and a decrease in arterial blood flow to the posterior temporal, occipital and parietal lobes, bilaterally (Josephs et al., 2006). Tsai et al. (2011) identified two variants of PCA, one impairing functions of the dorsal visual pathway leading to visual disorientation, Balint syndrome, and akinetopsia; the other variant leading to dysfunction of the ventral visual pathway where symptoms include visual agnosia, achromotopsia, prosopagnosia, and pure alexia. The authors conclude that with progression of PCA, the symptoms of these two variants do not overlap, but remain discrete.

Some subjects with PCA have visual hallucinations, while others do not. In a survey of 59 patients with the diagnosis of PCA, Josephs et al. (2006) found visual hallucinations in 13 subjects. This subset of patients, unlike the other 46 subjects studied, had MRI evidence of significant gray matter atrophy in the primary visual cortex, thalamus and hypothalamus, head of caudate nucleus, globus pallidus, putamen, and midbrain, with some atrophy in the basal forebrain. Because of the evolution of visual impairments in these 13 patients, including the emergence of visual hallucinations, the authors suggest that some subjects in the later stages of PCA fall under the category of *Lewy body dementia*. Lewy body dementia is characterized by fluctuating cognition, impaired activities of daily living, sleep disturbance, visuospatial difficulties (i.e., discrimination of size and form), attentional problems, and visual hallucinations (Possin, 2010). Subjects may also have difficulty copying, counting visual forms, and distinguishing overlapping figures (Mori et al., 2000; Papagno, 2002).

Progressive Alexia

Progressive alexia, an acquired peripheral reading disorder, is often the first clinical sign of posterior cortical atrophy (Benson, Davis, & Snyder, 1988; McMonagle, Deering, Berliner, & Kertesz, 2006). The various types of acquired reading disorders found in PCA include neglect alexia, alexia due to simultanagnosia, attentional alexia, and alexia due to progressive impairment in recognition of letter and word forms, characterized by letter-by-letter reading (Wilson et al., 2013).

REFERENCES

Barnes, D. & McDonald, W.I. (1992). The ocular manifestations of multiple sclerosis: 2. Abnormalities of eye movements. *Journal of Neurology, Neurosurgery & Psychiatry, 55*, 863-868.

Benson, D. F., Davis, R. J., & Snyder, B. D. (1988). Posterior cortical atrophy. *Archives of Neurology, 45*, 789-793.

Bhatti, M. T., Schmalfuss, I. M., Williams, L., & Quisling, R. G. (2003). Peripheral third cranial nerve enhancement in multiple sclerosis. *American Journal of Neuroradiology, 24*, 1390-1395.

Cronin-Golomb, A., Corkin, S., & Growdonn, J. H. (1995). Visual dysfunction predicts cognitive deficits in Alzheimer's disease. *Optometry and Vision Science, 72*(3), 168-176.

Daniels, S. K. (2006). Neurological disorders affecting oral, pharyngeal swallowing, part 1: Oral cavity, pharynx and esophagus. *GI Motility*. Retrieved from https://www.nature.com/gimo/contents/pt1/full/gimo34.html

Dutton, G. N. (2003). Cognitive vision, its disorders and differential diagnosis in adults and children: Knowing where and what things are. *Eye, 17*, 289-304.

Edwards, J. D., Ross, L. A., Wadley, V. G., Clay, O. J., Crowe, M., Roenker, D. L., & Ball, K. K. (2006). The Useful Field of View Test: Normative data for older adults. *Archives of Clinical Neuropsychology, 21*(4), 275-286.

Gillen, G. (2009). *Cognitive and perceptual rehabilitation: Optimizing function*. St. Louis, MO: Mosby Elsevier.

Globe, L. I., Dais, P. H., Schoenberg, B. S., & Duvoisin, R. C. (1988). Prevalence and natural history of progressive supranuclear palsy. *Neurology, 38*(7), 1031-1034.

Greene, J. D. (2005). Apraxia, agnosias, and higher visual function abnormalities. *Journal of Neurology, Neurosurgery, and Psychiatry, 76*(Suppl. V), v25-v34.

Heathfield, K. W. (1973). Huntington's chorea: A centenary review. *Postgraduate Medical Journal, 49*, 32-45.

Jackson, G. R. & Owsley, C. (2003). Visual dysfunction, neurodegenerative diseases, and aging. *Neurologic Clinics of North America, 21*, 709-729.

Josephs, K. A., Whitwell, J., Boevev, B. F., Knopman, D. S., Tang-Wai, D. F., Drubach, D. A., ... Peterson, R. C. (2006). Visual hallucinations in posterior cortical atrophy. *Archives of Neurology, 63*, 1427-1432.

Laatu, S., Revonsuo, A., Hamalainen, P., Ojanen, V., & Ruutiainen, J. (2001). Visual object recognition in multiple sclerosis. *Journal of Neurological Science, 185*, 77-88.

Lauterbach, E. C., Cummings, J. L., Duffy, J., Coffey, C. E., Kaufer, D., Lovell, M., ... Salloway, S. P. (1998). Neuropsychiatric correlates and treatment of lenticulostriatal disease: a review of the literature and overview of research opportunities in Huntington's, Wilson's, and Fahr's diseases. *Journal of Neuropsychiatry and Clinical Neuroscience, 10*, 249-266.

McMonagle, P., Deering, F., Berliner, Y., & Kertesz, A. (2006). The cognitive profile of posterior cortical atrophy. *Neurology, 66*, 331-338.

Mittenberg, W., Malloy, M., Petrick, J., & Knee, K. (1994). Impaired depth perception discriminates Alzheimer's dementia from aging and major depression. *Archives of Clinical Neuropsychology, 9*, 71-79.

Mittenberg, W., Choi, E. J., & Apple, C. C. (2000). Stereoscopic visual impairment in vascular dementia. *Archives of Clinical Neuropsychology, 15*(7), 561-569.

Mori, E. T., Shimomura, T., Fujimori, M., Hirono, N., Imamura, T., Hashimoto, M., … Hanihara, T. (2000). Visual-perceptual impairment in dementia with Lewy bodies. *Archives of Neurology, 57*, 489-493.

Mort, D. & Kennard, C. (2000). Adult neuro-degenerative diseases and their neuro-phthalmological features. *Optometry Today, 2*(Part 7), 33-37.

Paivio A. (1986). *Mental representations: A dual-coding approach.* New York, NY: Oxford University

Papagno, C. (2002). Progressive impairment of constructional abilities: A visuospatial sketchpad deficit? *Neuropsychologia, 40*, 1858-1867.

Perez, F. M., Runkel, R. S., Lachmann, E. A., & Nagler, W. (1996). Balint's syndrome arising from bilateral posterior cortical atrophy or infarction: Rehabilitation strategies and their limitation. *Disability and Rehabilitation, 18*(6), 300-304.

Platel, H., Lambert, J., Eustache, F., Cader, B., Dary, M., Viader, F., & Lechevalier, B. (1993). Characteristics and evolution of writing impairment in Alzheimer's disease. *Neuropsychologia, 31*, 1147-1158.

Possin, K. (2010). Visual spatial cognition in neurodegenerative disease. *Neurocase, 16*(6), 466-487.

Rehmann, H. U. (2000). Progressive supranuclear palsy. *Postgraduate Medical Journal, 76*, 333-336.

Rizzo, M., Anderson, S. W., Dawson, J., & Nawrot, M. (2000). Vision and cognition in Alzheimer's disease. *Neuropsychologia, 38*(12), 162-178.

Roh, H. S., Lee, S. Y., & Yoon, J. S. (2011). Comparison of clinical manifestations between patients with ocular myasthenia gravis and generalized myasthenia gravis. *Korean Journal of Ophthalmology, 25*(1), 1-7.

Sanders, A. F. (1970). Some aspects of the selective processing functional visual field. *Ergonomics, 13*(1), 101-117.

The National Institute of Neurological Disorders and Stroke (NINDS) 2018. https://www.ninds.nih.gov/Disorders/ Patient-Caregiver-Education/Hope-Through-Research/Parkinsons-Disease-Hope-Through-Research

Tsai, P.-H., Teng, E., Liu, C., & Mendez, M. F. (2011). Posterior cortical atrophy: Evidence for discrete syndromes of early-onset Alzheimer's disease. *American Journal of Alzheimer's Disease and Other Dementias, 26*(5), 413-418.

Warrington, E. K. & James, M. (1991). *The Visual Object and Space Perception Battery.* Bury St. Edmonds, United Kingdom: Thames Valley Test Company.

Weintraub, S. & Mesulam, M.M. (1988). Visual hemispatial inattention: Stimulus parameters and exploratory strategies. *Journal of Neurology, Neurosurgery and Psychiatry, 51*(12), 1481-1488.

Wilson, S.M., Rising, K., Stib, M.T., Rapcsak, S.Z., and Beeson, P.M. (2013). Dysfunctional visual word form processing in progressive alexia. *Brain, 136*(4), 1260-1273.

Test Bank Answer Key

CHAPTER 1

1. The ability to locate objects in space requires the integration of visual input with sensory information from the _____ and _____ systems. (Select 1)
   a. proprioceptive, auditory
   b. sensory, vestibular
   c. vestibular, proprioceptive
   d. auditory, vestibular

2. When we localize a word in relation to other words in a sentence we are using a(n) _____ perspective. (Select 1)
   a. egocentric
   b. allocentric
   c. central
   d. peripheral

3. There are two types of photoreceptor cells in the outermost sensory layer of the retina. Color vision is dependent upon the response of _____ cells to the presence of bright light. _____ cells respond to low light and movement. (Select 1)
   a. rod, cone
   b. light, dark
   c. ciliary, retinal
   d. cone, rod

McMartin Heeringa, H. *The Visual Brain and Peripheral Reading and Writing Disorders: A Guide to Visual System Dysfunction for Speech-Language Pathologists.* (pp. 101-104).

4. The retina may be divided into three distinct areas. Visual images are the sharpest when they are fixated by the _____ or _____. (Select 1)

a. fovea, peripheral retina

b. parafovea, central retina

c. parafovea, peripheral retina

d. fovea, central retina

5. Four cranial nerves are involved with vision. They are (Select 1):

a. II (optic), IV (trochlear), VI (abducens), and VIII (acoustic)

b. II (optic), III (oculomotor), IV (trochlear), and VI (abducens)

c. III (oculomotor), VI (abducens), V (trigeminal), and XI (accessory)

d. I (olfactory), II (optic), III (oculomotor), and IV (trochlear)

6. Visual input from the _____ retina is transmitted through the retinotectal pathway to the _____ in the brainstem. (Select 1)

a. peripheral, midbrain

b. peripheral, pulvinar

c. central, midbrain

d. central, pulvinar

7. The optic radiation is formed by neural fibers that represent the upper and lower visual fields. Neurons that represent the _____ visual field are in the _____ portion of the optic radiation. Neurons that represent the _____ visual field are in the _____ portion of the optic radiation. (Select 2)

a. peripheral, central

b. horizontal, lateral

c. upper, lower

d. lower, upper

8. The ventral visual pathway is also called the _____ because it carries information related to the detail of _____. The dorsal visual pathway is also called the _____ because it carries _____ and serves visually guided action. (Select 2)

a. "where" or "how" visual pathway, spatial information

b. "where" or "how" visual pathway, object information

c. "what" visual pathway, objects and faces

d. "what" visual pathway, facial information

9. The corpus callosum is a bundle of sensory nerve fibers that integrates the functions of the right and left hemispheres. Lesions of the corpus callosum may inhibit the transfer of information from the _____ hemisphere to the _____ hemisphere language areas. (Select 1)

a. left, right

b. right, left

c. left, right

d. right, right

10.There is a direct correspondence between points on the retina, layers of the lateral geniculate nucleus, points in primary visual cortex and divisions within the visual association cortex. This level of correspondence across structures and cortical locations that process visual information is called _____. (Select 1)

a. topographic organization

b. retinotopic organization

c. tonotopic organization

d. visual spatial organization

CHAPTER 2

1. When we read, words to the right of the fixation point are viewed with the _____ in order to plan the next rightward eye movement. (Select 1)

a. peripheral retina

b. central retina

c. parafoveal retina

d. bipolar retina

2. Normal aging effects on the visual system include: (Select all that apply)

a. reduced contrast sensitivity

b. reduced visual processing speed

c. decline in visual search ability

d. reduction in the Useful Field of View

3. Vision specialists who typically assess and treat visual motor and visual sensory deficits directly following brain injury and stroke include: (Select all that apply)

a. ophthalmologists

b. occupational therapists

c. speech language pathologists

d. behavioral or neurooptometrists

4. The eye movements that serve object recognition, reading and writing include: (Select 1)

a. contrast sensitivity, spatial orientation, fixation, and retinotopic organization

b. peripheral vision, accommodation, spatial orientation, and fixation

c. fixation, saccades, vergence, and accommodation

d. contrast sensitivity, saccades, retinotopic organization and fixation

5. Two types of visual motor disorders are characteristic of bilateral occipitoparietal lesions. _____ affects motor planning and eye-hand coordination when reaching for objects such as a pencil or word cards, while _____ affects the ability to gaze shift toward a new target outside the central retinal field. (Select 1)

a. optic ataxia, oculomotor apraxia

b. verbal apraxia, optic ataxia

c. oculomotor apraxia, optic ataxia

d. hemianopia, hemispatial neglect

6. _____ is a visual sensory impairment that prevents the reader from seeing whole words and interferes with the guidance of eye movements for reading. (Select 1)

a. peripheral retinal field loss

b. parafoveal field loss

c. upper visual field loss

d. contrast sensitivity

7. Subjects who have experienced a left hemisphere stroke may demonstrate right hemispatial neglect.

___ **True**

___ False

8. _____ affects reading and writing when it results in the inability to recognize number, letter and word forms. (Select 1)

a. optic ataxia

b. visual agnosia

c. visual motor impairment

d. gaze apraxia

9. Readers will use the "letter-by-letter" reading strategy when they: (Select 1)

a. have difficulty remembering what they just read

b. have difficulty matching sounds with letters

c. have hemispatial neglect

d. have difficulty recognizing letter and word forms due to visual agnosia

10. A referral to occupational therapy for visual system testing should be initiated: (Select all that apply)

a. when the client forgets to bring her glasses to speech therapy

b. when error patterns on reading and writing tests/exercises show signs of visual system dysfunction (e.g. hemispatial neglect, letter duplication errors, writing uphill or downhill)

c. when a client complains of visual changes post stroke or brain injury

d. when reading is impaired due to receptive aphasia

Index

McMartin Heeringa, H. *The Visual Brain and Peripheral Reading and Writing Disorders: A Guide to Visual System Dysfunction for Speech-Language Pathologists*. (pp. 105-109).
© 2019 Taylor & Francis Group.

Printed in the United States
by Baker & Taylor Publisher Services